Emergency Radiology

Rules and Tools

Published by the REMEDICA Group

REMEDICA Publishing Ltd., 32–38 Osnaburgh Street, London, NW1 3ND, UK

REMEDICA Inc, Tri-State International Center, Building 25, Suite 150, Lincolnshire, IL 60069, USA

E-mail: books@remedica.com

www.remedica.com

Publisher: Andrew Ward

In-house editors: Helen James and Emma Hawkridge

Design: Endre Buzogány

ISBN 1 901346 28 5

British Library Cataloguing-in Publication Data

A catalogue record for this book is available from the British Library

Printed and bound at Ajanta Offset & Packaging Ltd., India

Emergency Radiology
Rules and Tools

Elizabeth Dick
Ian Francis
Ian Renfrew

Editor:
Jane Young

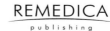
REMEDICA
p u b l i s h i n g

LONDON • CHICAGO

Acknowledgements and Dedications

Many thanks to Dr Otto Chan.
Dedicated to M & D, my inspiration as parents and doctors.

Elizabeth Dick

Many thanks to Dr Nic Bowley (Queen Victoria Hospital, East Grinstead)
for his support and allowing us access to his collection of images of maxillo-facial trauma.
Dedicated to Megan, William and Kitty.

Ian Francis

Many thanks to those who have educated us.
Dedicated to Angela and our families.

Ian Renfrew

Contents

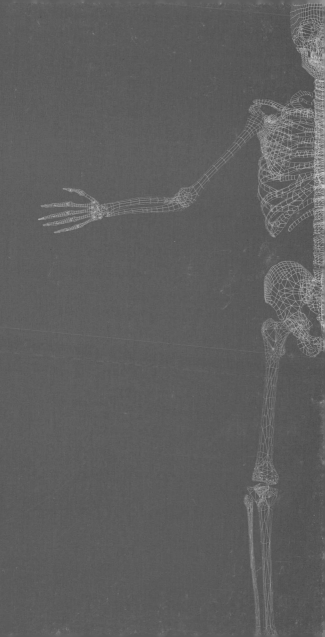

Contributors

Dr Elizabeth Dick, BSc, MBBS, MRCP, FRCR

Consultant Radiologist
St Mary's Hospital
London
UK

Dr Ian Francis, BDS (Hons), MBBS, FRCS, FRCR

Consultant Radiologist
Brighton and Sussex University Hospital
Brighton
UK

Dr Ian Renfrew, MBBS (Hons), MRCP, FRCR

Specialist Registrar in Radiology
Middlesex Hospital, UCLM NHS Trust
London
UK

Dr Jane Young, MBBS, MSc, FRCR (Editor)

Consultant Radiologist and Director of Medical Education
Whittington Hospital
London
UK

Foreword

Numerous health professionals including house officers, senior house officers (SHOs) and specialist registrars (SpRs) in training, and medical students are involved in the management of patients presenting in the Accident and Emergency (A&E) department. The volume of medical knowledge necessary to manage these patients can be overwhelming as virtually any medical condition can present itself in A&E. It is unfortunate that these patients are almost invariably seen initially by relatively inexperienced SHOs who must decide on the initial management pathways. Radiographs of these patients are ordered and the SHOs are left to interpret the radiograph without assistance. To compound all of these problems, these doctors have rarely received guidance – at medical school or during the SHO training – on how to interpret the radiographs. The radiographs often provide the only clue to the problem and may be the key to correct management of the patient.

With this in mind, the authors of *Emergency Radiology: Rules and Tools* have made a huge effort to provide a very simple step-by-step approach to interpreting radiographs, using clearly illustrated diagrams in addition to labeled radiographs, so that the reader can evaluate the radiograph systematically. The diagrams and radiographs are of an excellent quality and the comprehensible drawings make this a straightforward and easy book to read.

The book is very well laid out and is divided into anatomical regions; each chapter begins with a 'rules and tools' section and ends with a series of case studies. These case studies not only allow the reader to test their basic principles and knowledge of everyday conditions but also provide more difficult cases, which illustrate the common pitfalls that can occur when making a diagnosis.

Therefore, it is a privilege and a great pleasure to have been asked to write the foreword to this very original, new book. I am certain that it will be extremely popular, not only with SHOs and SpRs in A&E but also with medical students; house officers and SpRs in other specialties (e.g. orthopedics and radiology); and numerous other health professionals—in particular nurses and radiographers.

At present, litigation costs are escalating in the medical health profession. Using this book and the red dot system; examining the patients clearly and documenting the findings carefully; and rapid prioritised reporting of A&E radiographs should help to limit the number of mistakes that are made.

Dr Otto Chan
Consultant Radiologist
The Royal London Hospital, UK

Introduction

So here you are in the middle of the night with an X-ray that you are not sure about. What are you going to do?

Basic common sense

From the clinical examination you have taken, use what you have learned to decipher what the mechanism of injury is in each case. Share this information with the radiographer and radiologist to ensure that they provide you with the correct films and most helpful report. Deciphering the mechanism of injury will also help you to look at the X-ray. If the force or type of injury is very likely to have produced a fracture, then worry if you cannot see one. Ask someone else for their opinion, i.e. a radiographer, A&E registrar, consultant, nurse practitioner, radiologist, or orthopedic surgeon.

When it comes to children, listen to what they tell you (they are very sensible) and listen to their parent or carer. Check who was with them at the time of the incident and make sure you know the story and that it fits!

Adequate X-rays

It is crucial to visualize certain areas more than others, e.g. it is particularly important to visualize the cervical spine as far as C7/T1. Two views are essential, usually at 90° to each other, otherwise pathology can be easily missed.

If you are concerned about the quality of the X-ray, discuss this with the radiographer. It may be that the patient is very difficult to image and the radiographer may be able to think of some other view to help you.

Tips to remember:

• Where there is one fracture near a joint, always take another X-ray to include the joints above and below the fracture, as there may be a dislocation or second fracture.

• Some injuries are frequently associated with pathology at more than one site. For example, a fall from height, which frequently causes calcaneal fractures, is also often associated with vertebral fractures (the force is transmitted vertically through the body).

• Comparison with 'normals' may help—is there another 'normal' film lying nearby? Take a look at Keats' *Atlas of Normal Roentgen Variants*. This contains thousands of examples of appearances that seem to be within normal range, but can often be mistaken for pathology. A list of the normal films that appear in *Emergency Radiology: Rules and Tools* can be found on page 207.

• In children, the developing skeleton can look very strange, and yet be entirely normal. What can you do? 'Keats' will be your first 'port of call'. Then, as before, ask people who know more than you do. Occasionally, and usually in desperation, a film of the 'other' side may be necessary; however, since this is additional radiation, it should not be your decision, but usually that of a radiologist. There are strict regulations governing exposure to radiation (Ionising Radiation Medical Exposure Regulations 'IRMER' —in the UK) to avoid unnecessary examinations.

When should you do a 'follow-up' film?

These are useful when the likelihood of a fracture is high, but one is not visible. Also, certain fractures are difficult to see initially, yet are crucial not to miss, e.g. a scaphoid fracture. Repeat the film and examination at 10 days after the injury, since at this stage, there will be resorption of the fracture margins that make the fracture easier to see. The exception to this being if the patient returns earlier with symptoms, in which case your threshold for repeat should be lower.

Emergency Radiology: Rules and Tools provides essential theory and a framework for approaching emergency X-ray reporting. Working through the detailed and comprehensive cases in this book should help you to gain confidence in your diagnostic skills.

Jane Young

Skull and Face

Rules and Tools

Introduction

The facial skeleton and skull are the primary site for injury in assaults and road traffic accidents (RTAs).

Facial injuries range from minor dento-alveolar damage to complicated comminuted fractures of the facial skeleton with associated airway problems. The following points outline the incidence and other aspects connected with facial fractures:

- there is a 20% incidence of associated facial injuries in patients presenting with cervical spine fractures; in such cases both these skeletal areas should be examined carefully
- the diagnosis of a facial fracture should raise the suspicion of an associated injury (as high as 30–50%)
- the overall incidence of facial fractures in children is low (<10%)
- the relative incidence of fractures of the facial skeleton is as follows:
  45% middle third
  35% mandible
  20% nasal bones

'Middle third' facial fractures

Patients with suspected middle third fractures have a high incidence of associated life-threatening injuries, which may affect the degree to which the facial injuries can be investigated.

- Le Fort fractures—these are complex fractures, which are classified into three groups (shown in Figure 1). They all involve relative areas of weakness and a partial or complete separation of the maxilla from the rest of the facial bones
- Nasal bone fractures—these are usually clinically obvious. Routine X-rays are not necessary, but are performed when corrective surgery is contemplated
- Zygomatic/malar fractures—the most common fracture of the facial skeleton is the 'tripod' or tri-malar fracture. This involves the zygomatic arch; the inferior orbital rim and lateral wall of the maxillary antrum; and separation of the zygomatico-frontal suture (Figure 2)
- Orbital 'blow-out' fractures are usually the result of a direct blow to the globe. The rim remains intact, but the transmitted force fractures the thin bones of the orbital floor. The orbital contents herniate through the fracture (causing the 'tear drop' appearance). If the extraocular muscles are involved, the patient may have diplopia on upward gaze (this can only be determined if examination of the eye is possible). CT scans are particularly helpful in this group
- Superior orbital rim fractures—these may be associated with frontal sinus fractures

Figure 1. Le Fort fractures.

a) Le Fort I: Alveolar separation (a transverse fracture separating the alveolar process from the maxilla).

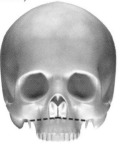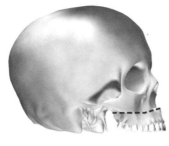

b) Le Fort II: Maxillary separation (a pyramidal fracture separating the central portion of the face).

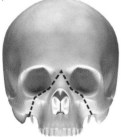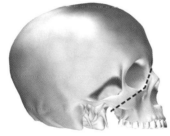

c) Le Fort III: Craniofacial separation (complete separation of the facial skeleton from the skull).

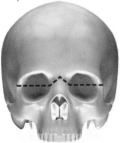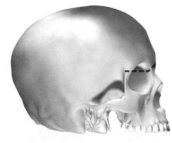

Figure 2. Tripod fracture.

The tripod fracture commonly consists of:
(1) separation of the zygomatico-frontal suture
(2) fracture of the zygomatic arch
(3) fracture of the inferior orbital rim extending through the anterior and lateral walls of the maxillary antrum

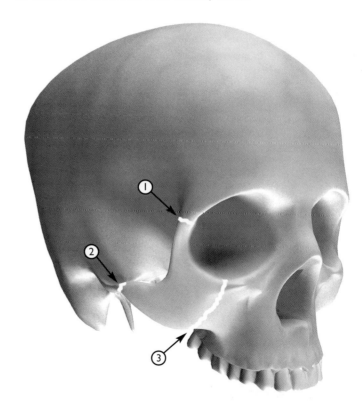

- Naso-ethmoidal fractures—these are usually the result of a direct blow to the nasion (bridge of nose), and frequently occur when the head hits the dashboard or steering wheel. All these bones are relatively thin, and are easily fractured and displaced. This is rarely an isolated injury and is mostly associated with multiple facial fractures. There may be an associated cerebrospinal fluid leak. There are several classifications of these injuries. Further evaluation is by CT

Middle facial bone views

- Occipitomental (OM)
- OM 30°
- Lateral
- Additional views include: Reverse Towne's (for the zygomatic arch)

Film-viewing routine

Look at:

- the maxillary sinus—a fluid level suggests a facial fracture, although commonly it can be a feature of sinusitis
- the orbital margins for fractures (see line 1, Figure 3)

- the orbits—the presence of air may indicate a sinus fracture, particularly of the frontal or ethmoid bone
- the 'elephant's trunk' of the zygomatic arch (see line 3, Figure 3)

When assessing each area, compare both sides looking for asymmetry.

Also look for:

- soft-tissue swelling
- a soft-tissue 'tear drop' from an inferior orbital margin indicating a 'blow-out' fracture (see line 2, Figure 3)

Figure 3. OM and OM 30°.
Line 1 indicates where to look for fractures of the orbital margins.
Line 2 indicates where to look for a soft-tissue 'tear-drop'.
Line 3 indicates where to look for discontinuity of the 'elephant's trunk' of the zygomatic arch.

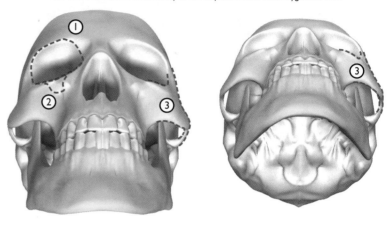

Figure 4. Distribution of fractures of the mandible. Multiple fractures occur in 50–60% of cases.

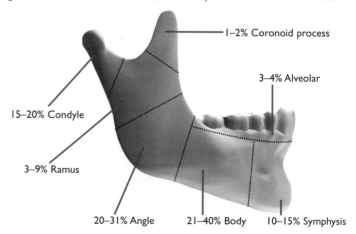

1–2% Coronoid process

3–4% Alveolar

15–20% Condyle

3–9% Ramus

20–31% Angle

21–40% Body

10–15% Symphysis

Dento-alveolar injury

Dental injuries involve the teeth with or without injury to the surrounding alveolar bone.

Dento-alveolar views
Two intra-oral views: peri-apical and upper/lower standard occlusal. An orthopantomogram (OPG) may be of use with posterior injuries. If part of a tooth is missing, it is vital that inhalation is excluded; thus a chest X-ray (CXR) is mandatory.

Film-viewing routine
Look for a fracture line, which is usually radiolucent in dento-alveolar injury. Occasionally it may be seen as a linear density due to overlapping of bony or apical fragments.

Mandibular fractures

Injuries of the mandible are best described and assessed, both clinically and radiographically, according to their anatomical site (Figure 4). The mandible can be subdivided into the following regions:
- the symphysis, which extends between the two canine teeth
- the body, which extends between the canine tooth anteriorly and the angle of the mandible posteriorly
- the ramus, which lies between the angle and the base of the condylar and coronoid processes

The relative frequency of fractures at these sites is shown in Figure 4. Multiple fractures occur in 50–60% of cases.

Mandibular views
There are a large number of possible projections that can be used (Table 1), but two views at right angles is the ideal.

Film-viewing routine
Look for:
- a step deformity
- a radiolucent or radiopaque fracture line

Additional information
Mandibular fractures are 'unfavorable' or 'favorable' depending on whether the bony fragments are distracted or not (due to the direction of the fracture line and the muscle pull, Figure 5). This determines management and outcome.

Table 1. Common radiographic projections used for assessment of mandibular trauma.

Site of injury	Radiographic projection
Symphysis	Lower standard occlusal
	Oblique lateral
	Peri-apical films
Body	OPG
Angle	Oblique lateral
Ramus	Posteroanterior (PA) mandible
Condyle	OPG
	Oblique lateral
	PA mandible
	Reverse Towne's
Coronoid process	OPG
	Oblique lateral
	OM

Figure 5. Favorable/unfavorable mandibular fractures.

a) Favorable fracture—muscle pull producing apposition of bony fragments.

b) Unfavorable fracture—muscle pull distracting bony fragments.

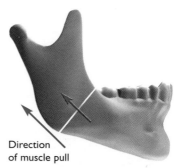

Direction of muscle pull

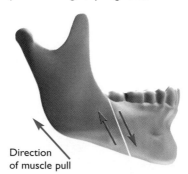

Direction of muscle pull

Skull vault and cranial base fractures

The value of skull X-rays for head injury is a controversial issue, with differing policies between institutions. The presence of a depressed skull fracture on X-ray is associated with a 33% chance of having a dural tear. A patient with neurological signs or impaired consciousness will need a CT scan, therefore skull X-rays are redundant. The history and site of injury are crucial pieces of information for aiding interpretation.

Skull views
- Anteroposterior (AP) or posteroanterior (PA)
- Lateral
- Towne's

Film-viewing routine
Look at:
- the upper cervical spine, particularly the atlanto-axial region for cervical spine injuries (see cervical spine section)
- the cortex of the skull vault in each projection—run your eye around it looking for discontinuity, as this may indicate a fracture

Look for:
- a fluid level in the sphenoid sinus on the lateral view—this indicates a skull-based fracture (Figure 6)
- soft-tissue swelling

Most difficulties in diagnosing skull fractures are in differentiating vascular impressions and true fractures. Typically, fractures have the following features:
- the fractures are lucent and straight
- the fractures tend to be sharp and black in outline as they involve both inner and outer tables
- the fractures can cross suture lines
- the fractures do not taper uniformly

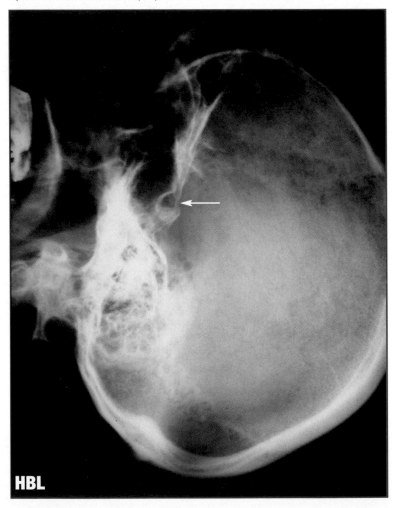

Figure 6. Air-fluid level sphenoid sinus indicated by an arrow. In cases of trauma, the patient is placed supine and a horizontal beam lateral (HBL) film is taken to check for an air-fluid level.

To ensure correct interpretation, knowledge of other lucencies in the skull is essential; they include:

- sutures and vascular grooves—these are usually curvilinear or tortuous, and the margins are not as sharp
- accessory sutures—these can be confusing, and are commonly seen in children. They may be unilateral and can be mistaken for fractures. The commonest is the metopic suture. If in doubt, Keats' *Atlas of Normal Roentgen Variants* has many examples

For normal skull radiographs, see Figures 7, 8, 9 and 10.

Figure 7. Normal AP skull.

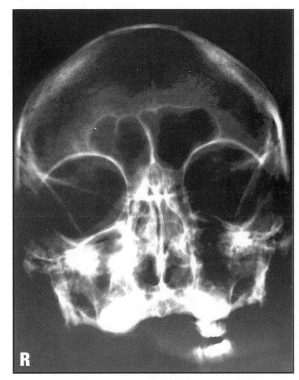

Figure 8. Normal Towne's view.

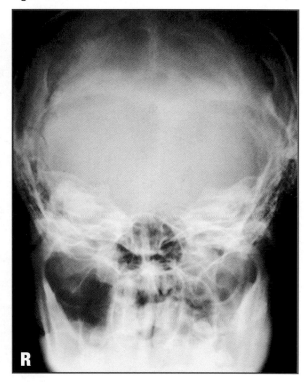

Additional information

- 80% of vault fractures are linear (well-defined radiolucent line)
- 15% of skull fractures are depressed fractures and most are within the frontoparietal region

Also, if **any** of the following features are seen on a child's X-ray, there is a possibility of non-accidental injury (NAI) and this **must** be taken seriously:

- occipital fractures (most pediatric fractures involve the parietal bone)
- fractures that cross a suture
- widely separated margins
- comminuted (i.e. non-linear) fractures

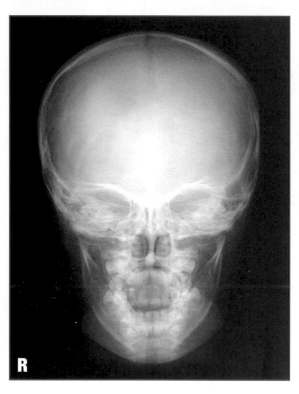

Figure 9. Normal AP skull in a child showing sagittal and lambdoid sutures.

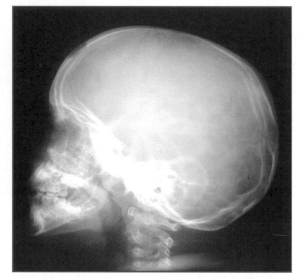

Figure 10. Normal lateral skull in a child showing coronal, lambdoid and accessory sutures.

Case Studies

Case 1

Clinical details

This seventeen-year-old male was hit in the face with a cricket ball.

Figure 1. OM 30°.

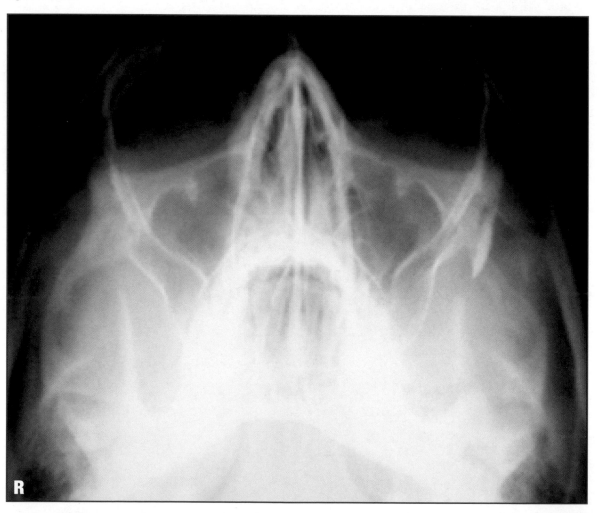

Radiological features

There is increased bony density in the region of the left zygomatic arch due to overlapping bone, with a loss in the normal arch contour. In addition, there is a horizontal lucency of the base of the left coronoid process.

Diagnosis

Fracture of the left zygomatic arch and left coronoid process of the mandible.

Discussion

The fractures are indicated on the OM 30° view opposite (Figure 2).

Figure 2. The OM 30° view with the fractures indicated.

1. fracture of the left zygomatic arch.
2. fracture of the left coronoid process.
3. normal right zygomatic arch.

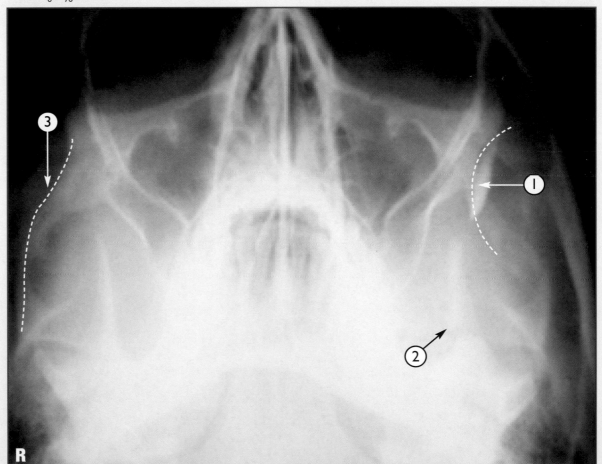

Case 2

Clinical details
This twenty-eight-year-old male
was involved in a drunken fight.

Figure 1. The OPG.

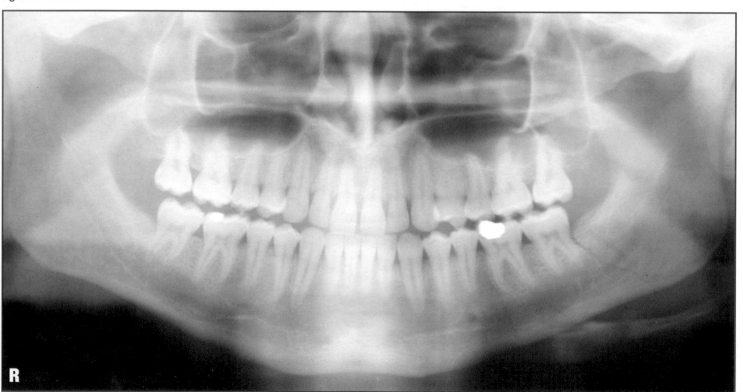

Radiological features

There is an irregular lucency in the region of the left angle of the mandible that involves the periodontal ligament of the lower left wisdom tooth.

Diagnosis

Fracture of the left angle of the mandible involving the lower left wisdom tooth.

Discussion

The fracture can be seen clearly on the OPG (Figure 2). On occasions, lateral oblique views of the mandible may be necessary.

Figure 2. The OPG with the fracture outlined.

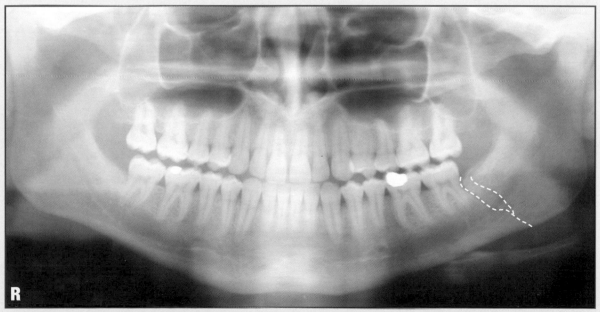

Case 3

Clinical details

This eighteen-year-old male was
involved in a fight—he complained
that his teeth did not 'bite' normally.

Figure 1. PA mandible.

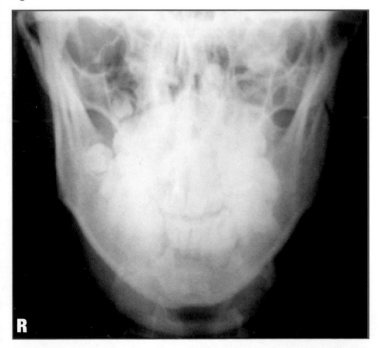

Figure 2. Left oblique mandible.

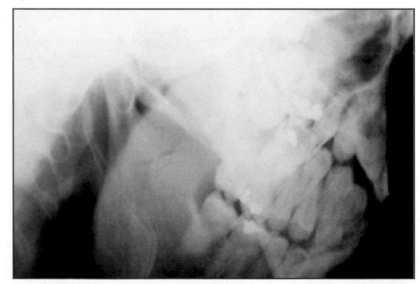

Radiological features

There is a linear lucency of the right body of the mandible involving several teeth. In addition, there is an associated lucency through the lower neck of the left condyle.

Diagnosis

Right body fracture of the mandible with associated left condylar neck fracture.

Discussion

The fractures are outlined on the PA and left oblique views below (Figures 3 and 4, respectively).

Figure 3. The PA view with the right body fracture and left condylar neck fracture outlined.

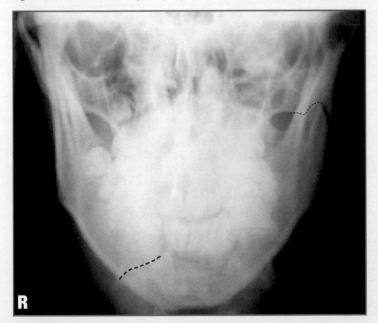

Figure 4. The left oblique view with the left condylar neck fracture outlined.

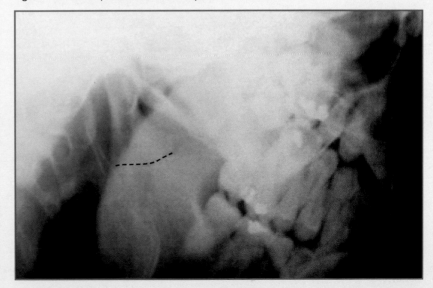

Case 4

Clinical details

This twenty-year-old male was assaulted—punched and kicked to the face.

Figure 1. The OPG.

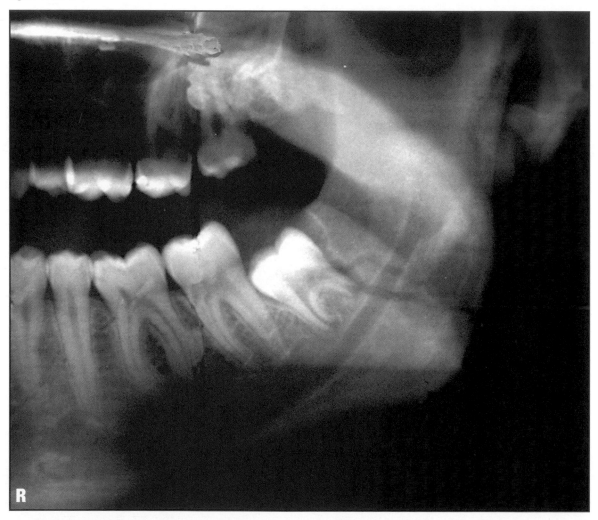

Radiological features

There is an irregular lucency involving the left angle of the mandible. This extends to involve the periodontal membrane of the wisdom tooth and crosses the inferior dental canal.

Diagnosis

Fracture of the left angle of the mandible.

Discussion

The fracture is outlined on the OPG opposite (Figure 2).

Figure 2. The OPG with the fracture outlined. The arrow indicates the alveolar canal.

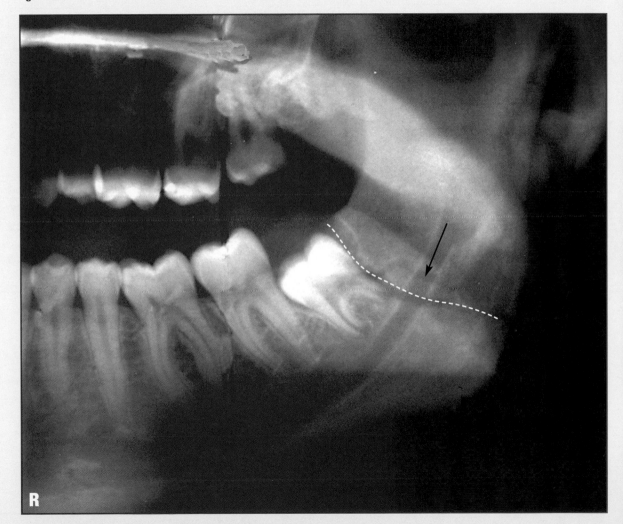

Case 5

Clinical details
This twenty-eight-year-old male was involved in an RTA and was found at the scene drunk and not wearing a seatbelt.

Figure 1. OM.

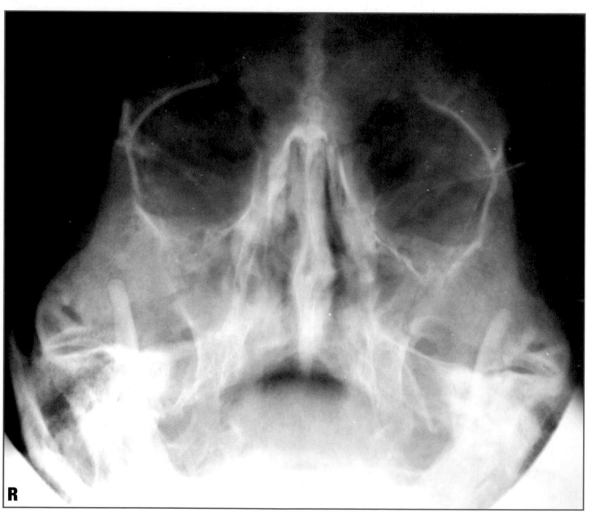

Radiological features

There is opacification of both maxillary antra and evidence of soft-tissue swelling. Bony continuity is lost in several sites, i.e. the lateral antral walls, inferior orbital margins and nasal bones.

Diagnosis

Le Fort II fracture of the middle third of the face.

Discussion

The Le Fort II fracture is outlined on the OM opposite (Figure 2).

Figure 2. OM.

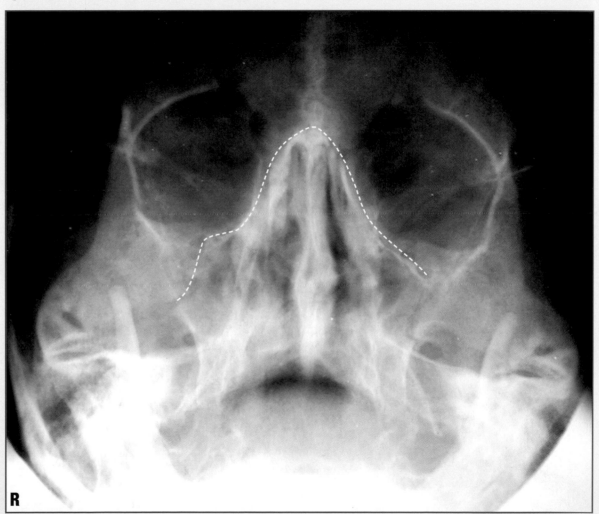

Case Studies

Case 6

Clinical details

This worker was hit by a metal pipe on a building site.

Figure 1. The OPG.

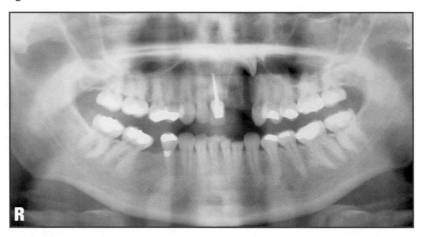

Figure 2. OM.

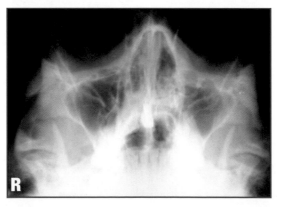

Figure 3. Upper standard occlusal and peri-apical view.

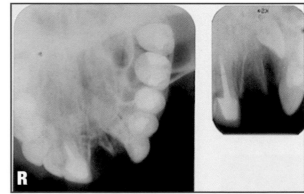

Radiological features

The upper left first and second incisors (L12) have been avulsed from their sockets. The upper left first incisor (L1) is not seen. The upper left second incisor (L2) is displaced superiorly and posteriorly into the junction of the hard palate and nasal spine, causing a fracture.

Diagnosis

Dento-alveolar injury with avulsion and displacement of teeth.

Discussion

Where teeth are missing either as a whole or in part, it is important to exclude inhalation. Thus, a CXR is mandatory. The displaced tooth is indicated on the OPG and OM views opposite (Figures 4 and 5, respectively).

Figure 4. The OPG with the dento-alveolar injury. L2 is indicated by an arrow.

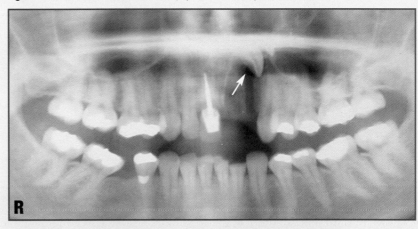

Figure 5. The OM view with the dento-alveolar injury. The displaced second incisor is outlined.

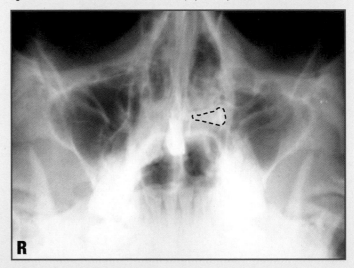

Case Studies

Case 7

Clinical details
This twenty-four-year-old male was
involved in a drunken brawl.

Figure 1. OM 30°.

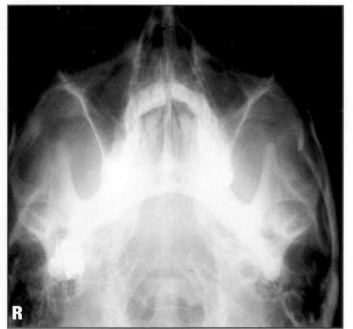

Figure 2. SMV.

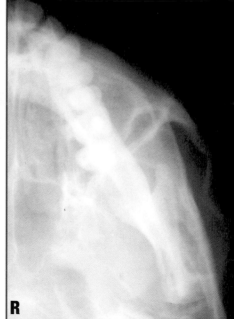

Radiological features

On the OM projection, there is an increased bony density overlying the left zygomatic arch and a loss of its normal configuration. The fracture and loss of normal arch contour are also visible on the submentovertical (SMV) projection.

Diagnosis

Depressed fracture of the left zygomatic arch.

Discussion

The features of the depressed zygomatic arch fracture are apparent on the OM film. An SMV view is rarely justified. Both views are shown below with the loss of normal arch contour outlined (Figures 3 and 4).

Figure 3. OM 30° with the loss of normal arch contour outlined.

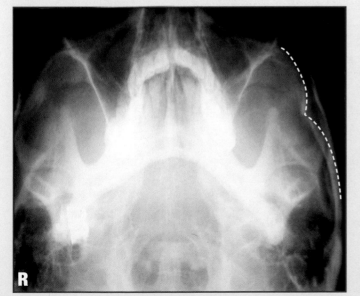

Figure 4. SMV with the loss of normal arch contour outlined.

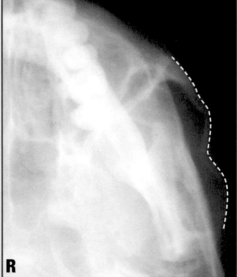

Case Studies

Case 8

Clinical details
This twenty-four-year-old soldier fainted whilst on parade ground duty.

Figure 1. Left oblique mandible.

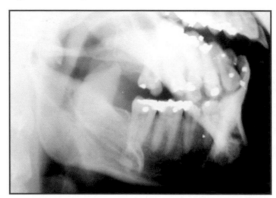

Figure 2. Right oblique mandible.

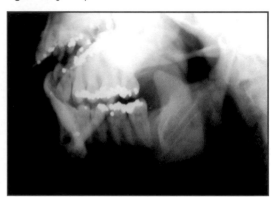

Figure 3. The OPG.

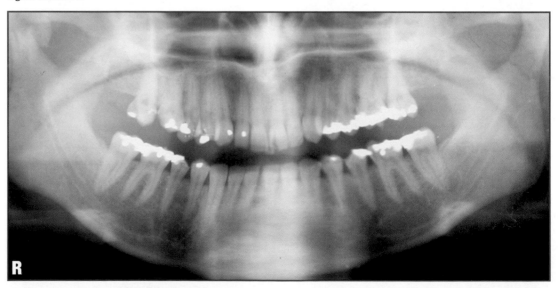

Radiological features

There is displacement of the right condylar head and a linear lucency involving the left condylar neck. There is also a suspicion of an irregular lucency through the right parasymphyseal region.

Diagnosis

Bilateral condylar fracture and associated parasymphyseal fracture (Guardsmen fracture).

Discussion

The Guardsmen fracture is outlined on the left oblique, right oblique and OPG views opposite (Figures 4, 5 and 6, respectively).

Figure 4. The left oblique view with the left condylar fractures outlined.

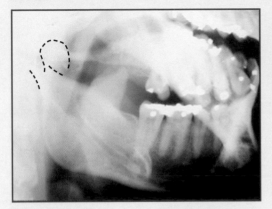

Figure 5. The right oblique view with the right condylar fracture outlined.

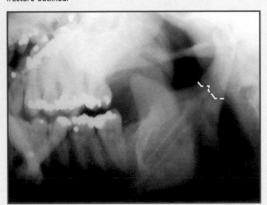

Figure 6. The OPG with the Guardsmen fracture outlined.

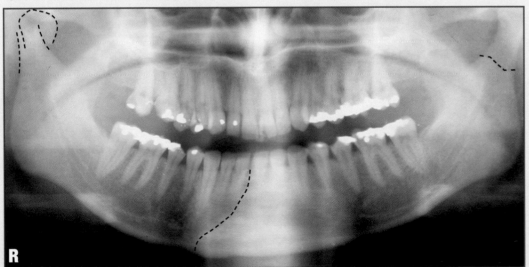

Case 9

Clinical details

This thirty-eight-year-old male
was involved in an RTA and
was not wearing a seat belt.

Figure 1. Lateral skull for soft-tissues.

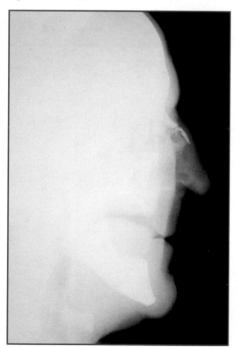

Figure 2. OM.

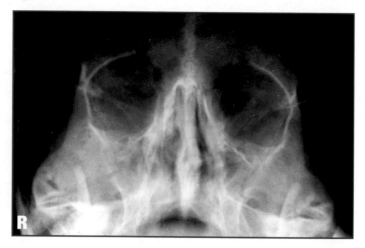

Figure 3. OM 30°.

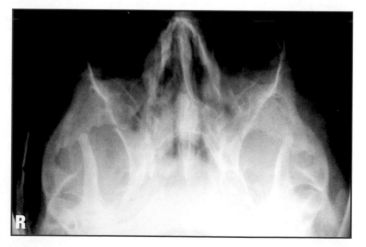

Radiological features

There is opacification of both maxillary antra associated with a pyramidal fracture of the middle third of the face. There is cortical interruption of the nasal bones (lateral projection); lateral wall of the nose; inferior orbital margins; and lateral antral walls.

Diagnosis

Le Fort II fracture.

Discussion

The Le Fort II fracture is outlined on the OM and OM 30° views below (Figures 4 and 5, respectively).

Figure 4. The OM with the Le Fort II fracture outlined.

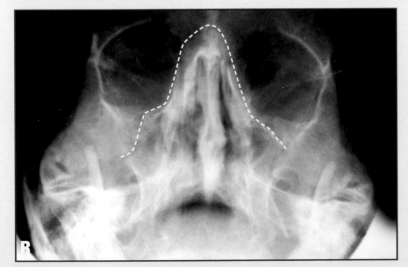

Figure 5. The OM 30° with the Le Fort II fracture outlined.

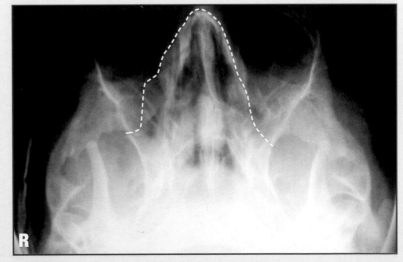

Case 10

Clinical details

This twenty-eight-year-old male was punched during a football match—he complained of blurred and double vision.

Figure 1. OM.

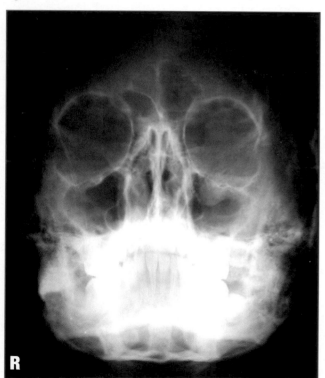

Figure 2. Tomographic view.

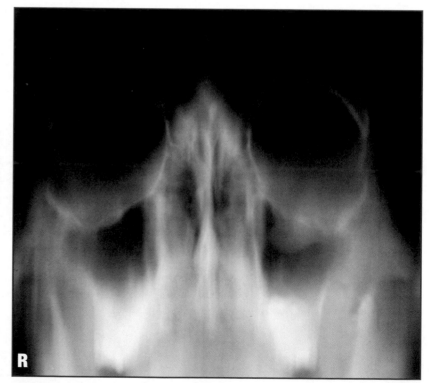

Radiological features

There is increased soft-tissue density within the superior aspect of the left maxillary antrum. There is also a linear density projected within the antrum that represents a displaced fragment of orbital floor.

Diagnosis

Left orbital blow-out fracture.

Discussion

This is the classical 'tear drop' fracture, as shown on the tomographic view. Typically a spicule of orbital floor acts as a trap door, which results in strangulation of small amounts of prolapsed orbital tissue. Coronal CT assessment is mandatory for treatment planning. The 'tear drop' fracture is outlined on the OM and tomographic views below (Figures 3 and 4, respectively).

Figure 3. The OM with the left 'tear drop' outlined.

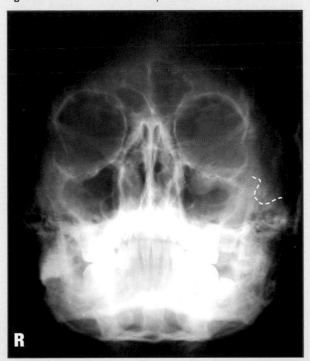

Figure 4. The tomographic view with the left 'tear drop' outlined.

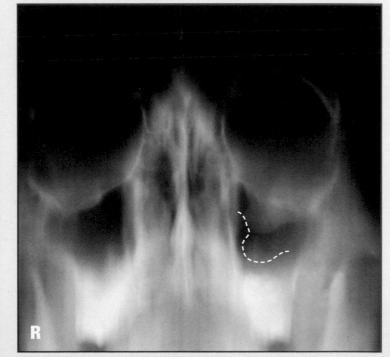

Case 11

Clinical details

This twenty-one-year-old male was elbowed playing football.

Figure 1. OM 30°.

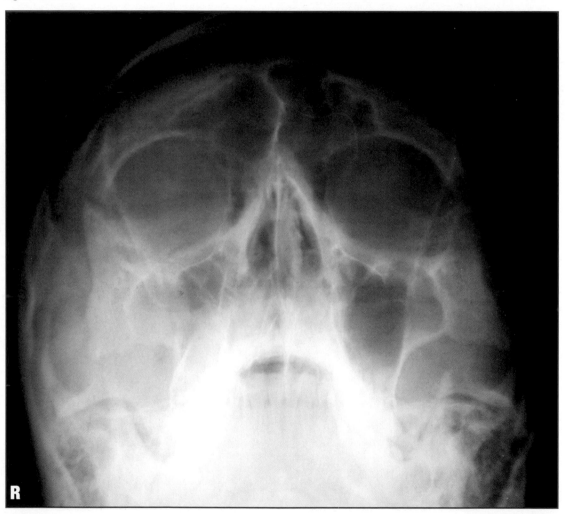

Radiological features

There is an air-fluid level in the right maxillary antrum. In addition, there is loss of continuity of bony outline involving the right lateral antral wall, right inferior orbital margin and right zygomatic arch. There is also widening of the right zygomatico-frontal suture.

Diagnosis

Right malar (tripod) fracture.

Discussion

The features of the right malar (tripod) fracture are outlined on the OM 30° view opposite (Figure 2).

Figure 2. The OM 30° with the fractures of the right malar (tripod) fracture outlined:
1. the air-fluid level in the right maxillary antrum
2. loss of continuity of bony outline of the right lateral antral wall
3. loss of continuity of bony outline of the right inferior orbital margin
4. loss of continuity of bony outline of the right zygomatic arch
5. widening of the right zygomatico-frontal suture.

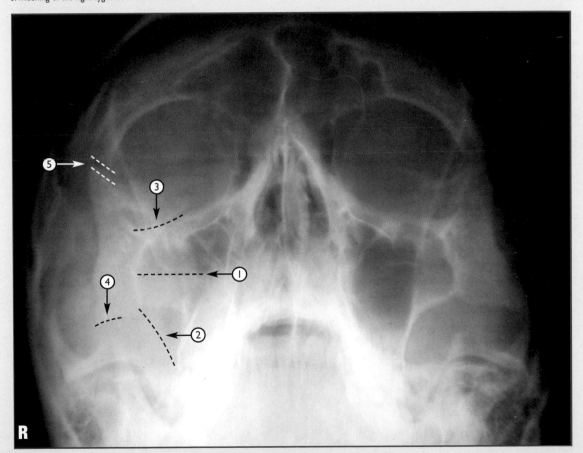

Case Studies

Case 12

Clinical details
This twenty-four-year-old male
was involved in a drunken fight.

Figure 1. OM 30°.

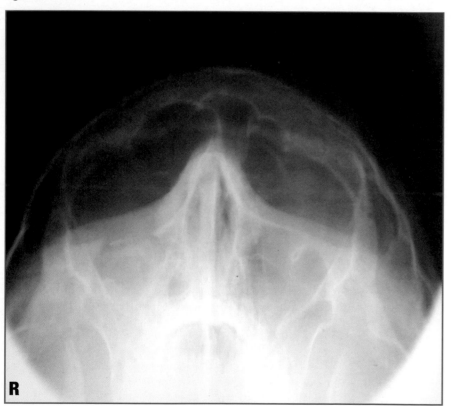

Radiological features
There is an obvious and complete
step deformity of the right
inferior orbital margin and an
increased density within the
right maxillary antrum.

Diagnosis
Depressed fracture of the right
inferior orbital rim.

Case 13

Clinical details

This twenty-four-year-old male was hit by a golf ball—he complained of double vision.

Figure 1. OM 30°.

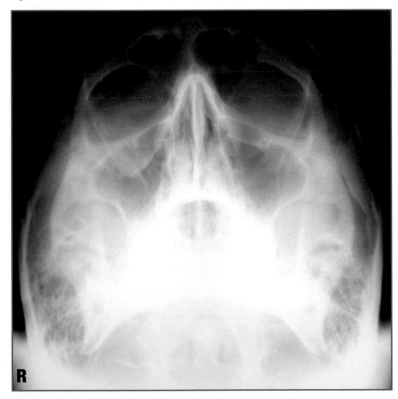

R

Radiological features

There is increased bony density in the right maxillary antrum. There is marked asymmetry between the right orbital floor and inferior right orbital rim when compared to the left.

Diagnosis

Right blow-out fracture.

Discussion

This is the more frequent appearance of a 'hammock type' blow-out fracture. The fracture is outlined on the OM 30° view below (Figure 2). CT examination is essential for treatment planning.

Figure 2. The OM 30° view with the fracture outlined.

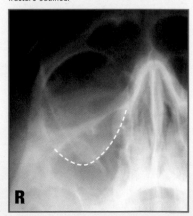

R

Case 14

Clinical details

This seventeen-year-old male was hit in the eye with a cricket ball.

Figure 1. OM.

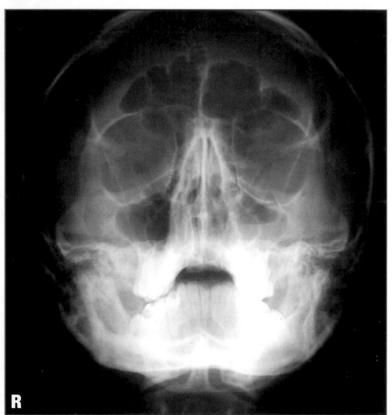

Radiological features

On the OM projection, there is a subtle discontinuity of the medial aspect of the left inferior orbital rim, and an air-fluid level in the left maxillary antrum.

Diagnosis

Fracture of the left inferior orbital rim.

Discussion

The step deformity is more obvious on the OM 30° projection as shown in Figure 2.

Figure 2. OM 30°.

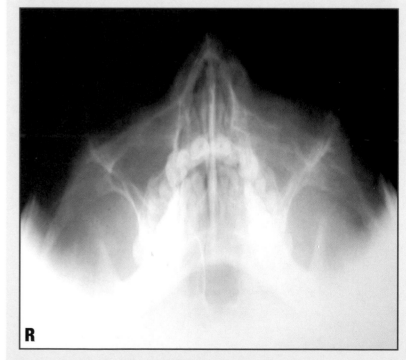

Case 15

Clinical details
This twenty-year-old male was assaulted with a baseball bat.

Figure 1. OM.

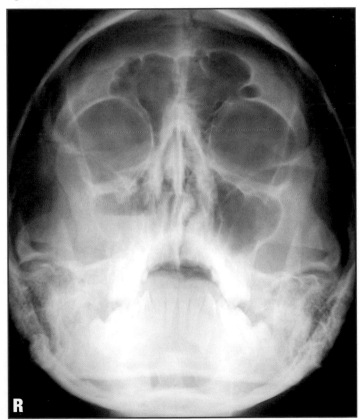

Radiological features
There is an air-fluid level within the right maxillary antrum. In addition, there is bony discontinuity of the lateral wall of the right maxillary antrum, the right inferior orbital margin and the right zygomatic arch. Abnormal alignment of the right zygomatico-frontal suture is also demonstrated.

Diagnosis
Right malar (tripod) fracture.

Discussion
The features of the right malar (tripod) fracture are outlined on the OM view below (Figure 2).

Figure 2. The OM view with the features of the right malar (tripod) fracture outlined:
1. air-fluid level within the right maxillary antrum
2. bony discontinuity of the lateral wall of the right maxillary antrum
3. bony discontinuity of the right inferior orbital margin
4. bony discontinuity of the right zygomatic arch
5. abnormal alignment of the right zygomatico-frontal suture.

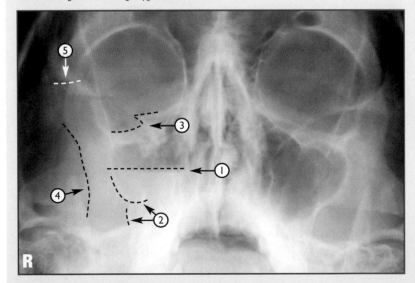

Case 16

Clinical details

This thirty-year-old male was assaulted and found on the roadside with a swollen right eye.

Figure 1. OM.

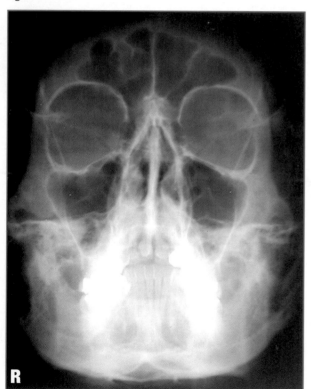

Figure 2. OM 30°.

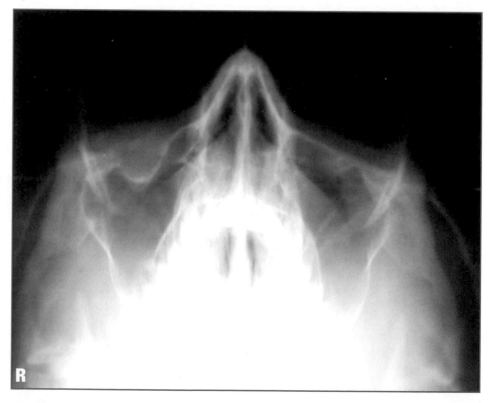

Radiological features

Subtle increase in bony density of the lateral aspect of the right inferior orbital rim is visible on the OM projection. On the OM 30° projection, displacement of the right inferior orbital rim is visible.

Diagnosis

Right inferior orbital rim fracture.

Discussion

The fracture, accompanying an increase in bony density, is indicated on the OM view opposite (Figure 3).

Figure 3. The OM view with the fracture (and increase in bony density) indicated by an arrow.

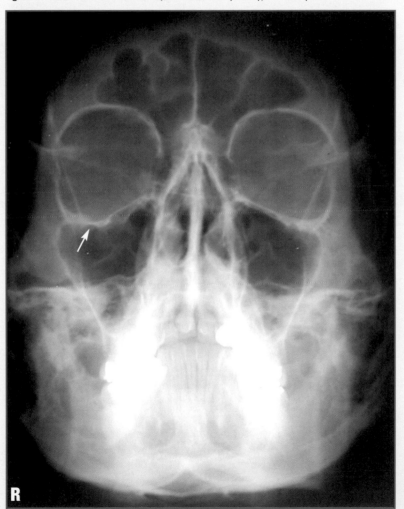

Case 17

Clinical details
Worried parents brought their child in after she fell off a table. Is there a fracture? Do you need other views?

Figure 1. Lateral skull.

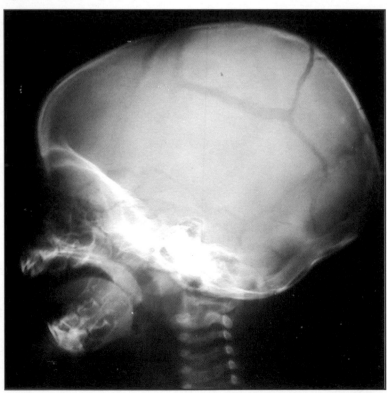

Radiological features
There is a comminuted fracture of the parietal bone.

Diagnosis
Comminuted fracture of parietal bone, suspicious of NAI.

Discussion
The fracture line is widely separated (>5 mm), a feature suggestive of NAI.

The other features of NAI are:
1. A comminuted or complex fracture
2. The fracture crosses a suture line (e.g. the lambdoid suture posteriorly)
3. A fracture of the occipital bone (not seen in this case)

The most common site for skull fractures in all children that are not due to NAI is the parietal bone. If there is a simple narrow (<5 mm) lucent fracture line in the parietal bone of a child with an appropriate history, then it can be considered to be non-suspicious.

Any possible NAI needs immediate referral to the pediatrician who will involve the child protection officer if necessary. Further investigation would include a cranial CT scan and skeletal survey. The latter should be requested by the pediatrician after the child has been assessed.

Important things to remember:
1. The history of the mechanism of injury should fit with the findings. In this case, falling off a table is rather minor trauma for the severity of the findings
2. The age of the child is important; check if he/she is old enough to roll, crawl, or walk. If not, the child may have been too young to roll off a surface, i.e. this is not the true story
3. Significant delay in bringing the child to A&E is suspicious and should warrant immediate pediatric referral

Case 18

Clinical details
This man was found unconscious at the bottom of the stairs after leaving his friends in a bar. He attended the Emergency Department with a severe headache.

Radiological features
AP and lateral skull show a bilateral parietal fracture.

Diagnosis
Bilateral parietal fracture.

Discussion
Patient needs referral to neurosurgery and a CT of the head if the Glasgow Coma Scale is reduced.

Figure 1. AP skull.

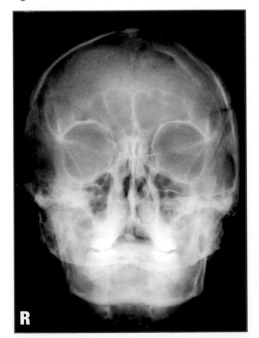

Figure 2. Lateral skull.

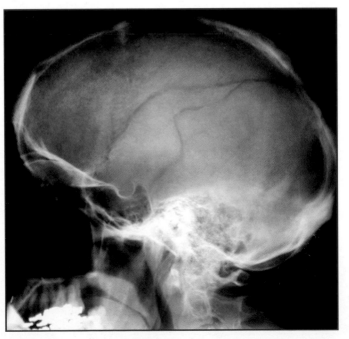

Case 19

Clinical details

This patient was playing rounders with his brother. The injury was unwitnessed, but his mother brought him to the Emergency Department.

Diagnosis

Depressed parietal right skull fracture.

Discussion

A CT of the head must be performed. The fracture is outlined on the lateral view below (Figure 2).

Figure 1. Lateral skull.

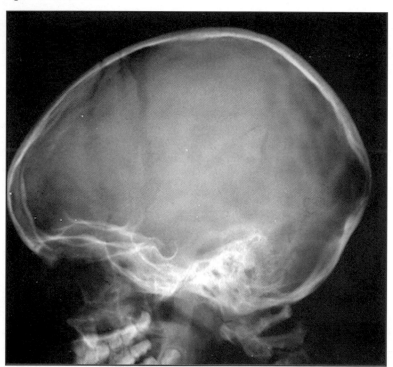

Figure 2. The lateral skull with the fracture outlined.

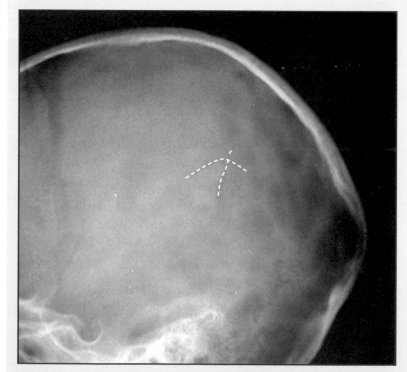

Case 20

Clinical details

This 18-month-old girl fell from her pushchair, which ran down ten stone steps. She suffered temporary loss of consciousness. She has vomited twice since the accident.

Figure 1. AP skull.

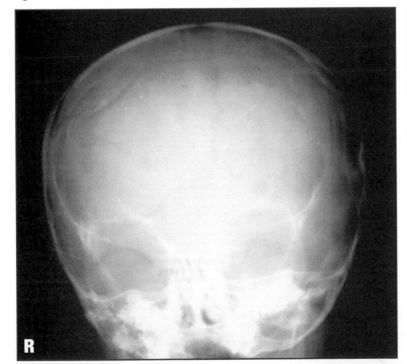

Radiological features/Diagnosis

There is a right temporo-parietal fracture which crosses the sagittal suture and extends into the left temporo-parietal bone.

Discussion

The patient needs to be admitted for observation. A CT of the head is required if the level of consciousness is reduced. The fracture is outlined on the AP view below (Figure 2).

Figure 2. The AP skull with the fracture outlined.

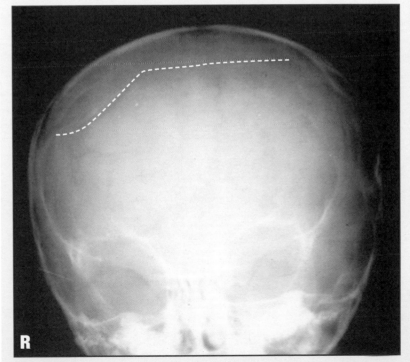

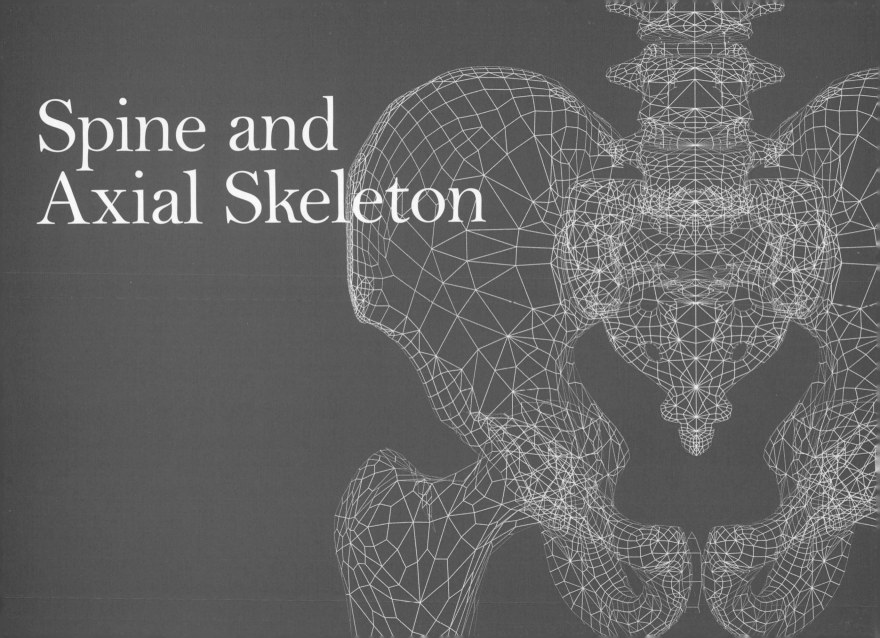

Spine and Axial Skeleton

Rules and Tools

Spine—Introduction

Spinal fractures may cause injury to adjacent neural structures at the time of the original insult. Careful handling and assessment of the patient is crucial to avoid neurological damage due to instability of bony and ligamentous structures.

Injuries of the spine are classified according to the following mechanisms:
- flexion injuries
- flexion and rotation injuries
- extension injuries
- compression injuries

The minimum imaging required are anteroposterior (AP) and lateral projections of the cervical, thoracic and lumbar regions of the spine. It is important to look at both the bones and soft-tissue regions on each view.

Cervical spine

Cervical spine injuries are serious and should all be treated initially as if they were unstable. Remember that, as well as the cord, structures surrounding the cervical spine may be damaged and these include: ligaments, emerging nerve roots, soft-tissues of the pharynx, the upper esophagus and carotid sheaths.

Cervical views
- Lateral (cranio-cervical junction to the upper border of T1)
- AP (mid and lower cervical region)
- AP 'peg' view of C1 and C2

Film-viewing routine

Lateral view (Figure 1)

Check the vertebral alignment using the anatomical lines below:

- anterior spinal line (ASL)—joins the anterior aspects of the vertebral bodies
- posterior spinal line (PSL)—joins the posterior aspects of the vertebral bodies
- spinolaminar line (SL)—joins the anterior margin of the 'junction of the laminae and spinous processes'
- posterior pillar line (PPL)—joins the posterior surface of the facet joints
- spinous line (SPL)—joins the tips of the spinous processes

Next:

- check each vertebral body in turn—their size and shape, and continuity between vertebral body and posterior elements
- check all facet joints are aligned
- look for pre-vertebral soft-tissue swelling (the normal pre-vertebral soft-tissue interval is <7 mm above C5 and <one vertebral body width below C5)

Don't forget to look for:

- fracture of the odontoid
- fracture of the C1 or C2 lamina
- posterior displacement of the posterior elements of C1 or C2 from the smooth arc of the SL—this indicates a Jefferson (C1) or Hangman's (C2) fracture
- widening of the atlanto-axial distance (normal measurements are 3 mm for adults and <5 mm for children)—this indicates rupture/laxity of the transverse ligament or fracture of the odontoid
- widening of the intervertebral disc spaces—this can occur with hyperextension injury and ligamentous rupture

Figure 1. Normal lateral radiograph of the cervical region of the spine.

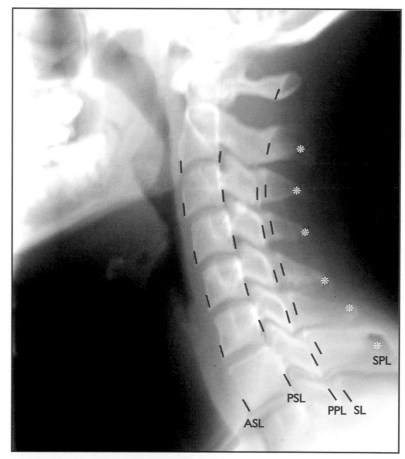

(ASL: anterior spinal line; PSL: posterior spinal line; PPL: posterior pillar line; SL: spinolaminar line; * = SPL: spinous line).

AP view (Figure 2)

Check:

- the spinous processes are in a straight line (Figure 2)—this straight line deviates in unilateral facet dislocation
- if the spinous processes are bifid—the line should run between them
- the distance between each spinous process is roughly equal—abnormal widening occurs in an anterior cervical dislocation or posterior ligament rupture (Figure 3)

Figure 2. Normal AP radiograph of the cervical region of the spine (∗ = spinous process).

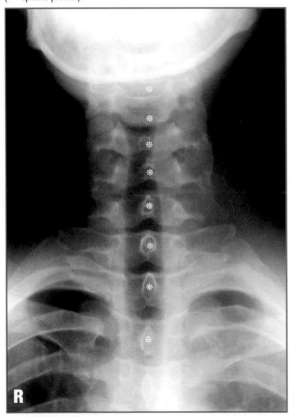

Figure 3. Abnormal widening of the interspinous distance—illustrated on the lateral view (top) and AP view (bottom).

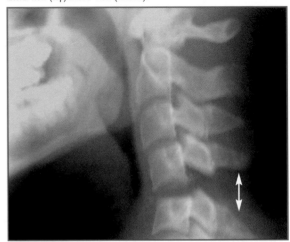

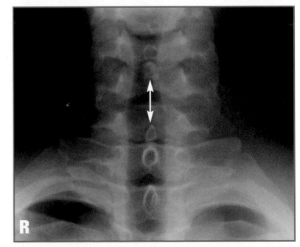

Open mouth 'peg' view (Figure 4)
Look:

- for a fracture of the odontoid peg
- at the lateral masses of C1—these should align with the lateral margin of C2 (see dashed white line, Figure 4)
- for asymmetry in the space between the odontoid peg and the lateral masses of C2 (for normal symmetrical space, see arrow heads, Figure 4)—this is difficult as asymmetry can appear due to rotation of the neck. However, it may mean there is a fracture of the 'ring' of the atlas (C1) with separation of the fragments

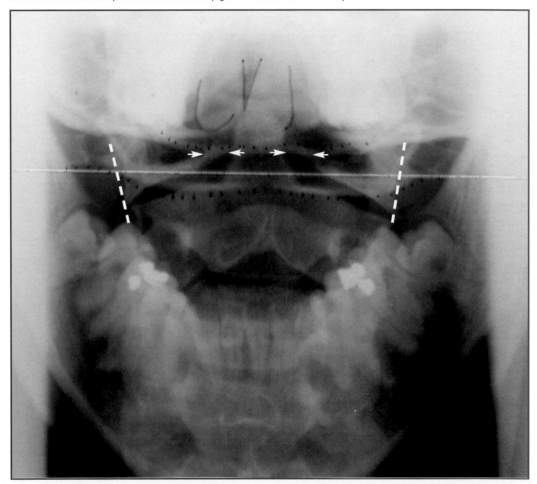

Figure 4. Normal open mouth 'peg' radiograph. The dashed lines show that the lateral masses of C1 and C2 are aligned. Arrow heads show that the space between the odontoid peg and the lateral masses of C2 is symmetrical.

Thoracic and lumbar spine

Denis' three-column theory of spinal stability

The spine is divided into anterior, middle and posterior columns:

- the anterior column includes: the anterior spinal ligament, the anterior intervertebral disc and the anterior part of the vertebral body
- the middle column includes: the posterior part of the vertebral body, the posterior intervertebral disc and the posterior longitudinal ligament
- the posterior column includes: the neural arch and all soft-tissue structures between the posterior elements

The middle column acts as a 'hinge' between the anterior and posterior column during flexion and extension.

In most spinal injuries, if the middle column is intact, the injury is stable, but if it is disrupted, the injury is unstable.

Figure 5. Denis' three-column theory of spinal stability. The three columns – posterior, middle and anterior – are outlined. The middle column functions as a fulcrum, and in flexion the anterior column is placed in compression and the posterior column in extension.
Reprinted from Rogers LF. Radiology of Skeletal Trauma. 3rd edition. Churchill Livingstone, 2001, with permission from Elsevier Science.

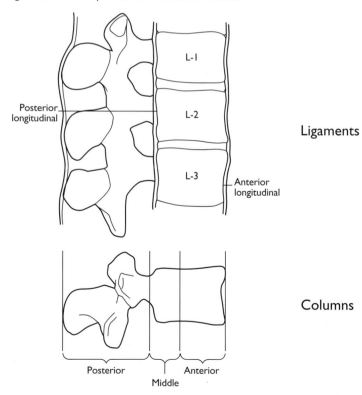

Thoracic and lumbar views

- AP
- Lateral

Film-viewing routine

AP view (Figures 6a and 6b)

Check:

- the paraspinal lines (Figure 6a)—widening implies local hemorrhage and possible spinal injury (Figure 6b)
- the lateral margins of the vertebral bodies—they should be aligned
- the contour of each vertebral body and its pedicles in turn—a fracture may be present, or loss of height or loss of symmetry

Figure 6. Assessment of the paraspinal lines from the AP view.

a) AP view of the chest with the normal paraspinal lines outlined.

b) AP view of the chest with the widening of paraspinal lines outlined.

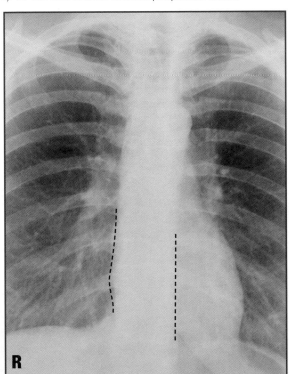

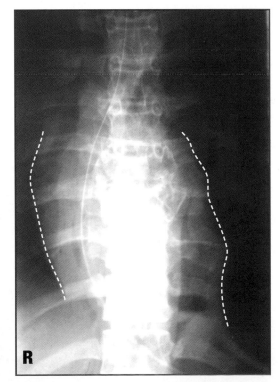

Lateral view (Figures 7a, 7b and 7c)
Check:

- vertebral alignment (Figure 7a) of the anterior, middle and posterior columns
- the height of the vertebral bodies and discs—single vertebral collapse causes a localized angulation (as shown in Figure 7b), whereas multilevel collapse of adjacent vertebrae causes a more gentle curvature (as shown in Figure 7c)

Figure 7. Assessment of the alignment of vertebral elements from the lateral view.

a) Lateral view of the normal alignment of vertebral elements.

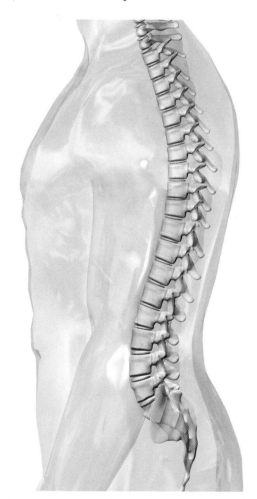

b) Lateral view of single vertebral collapse.

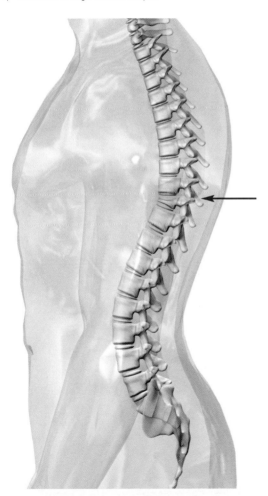

c) Lateral view of multilevel collapse of adjacent vertebrae.

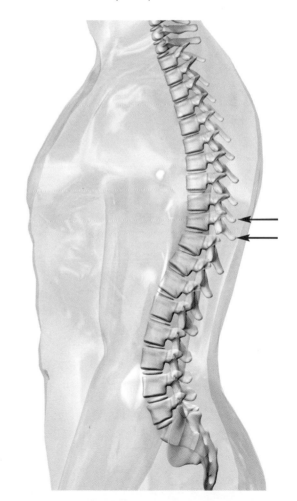

Additional information: stable and unstable fractures

Vertebral body fractures in isolation are generally stable, the exceptions being:

- burst fractures, which extend into the pedicles
- burst fractures with posterior displacement of fragments into the spinal canal (as the thoracic spinal canal is narrower than the lumbar spinal canal, it is particularly at risk from posterior protrusion of bone or disc)
- marked anterior vertebral collapse, which may be associated with interspinous ligament rupture (seen as widening of the interspinous interval posteriorly)

Stable and unstable vertebral fractures are shown in Figures 8 and 9 .

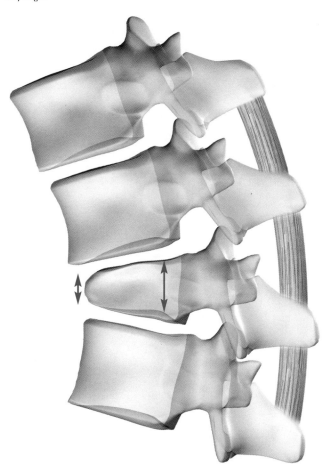

Figure 8. Stable wedge fracture with minor posterior vertebral bulge into canal. The ligaments are intact. However, there is decreased anterior and posterior vertebral body height.

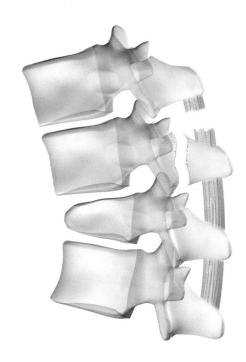

Figure 9. Unstable fractures.

a) A wedge fracture and avulsion fracture of the next superior spinous process with interspinous ligament rupture.

b) A wedge fracture with interspinous ligament rupture causing widening of the interspinous interval.

c) A wedge fracture with a bilateral fracture of the superior articular facets of the pars interarticularis and rupture of the interspinous ligaments. Note the anterior translocation of the superior vertebra.

d) Shearing force leading to vertebral fracture, anterior translocation of the superior vertebrae and rupture of the interspinous ligaments. Bilateral facet joint dislocation may be complicated by fracture.

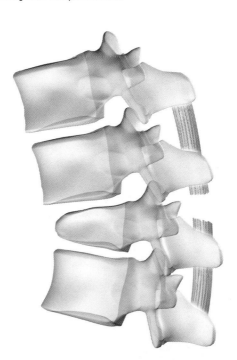

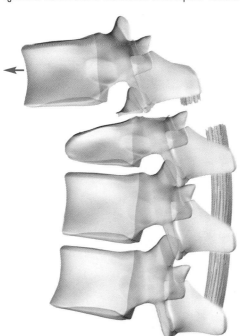

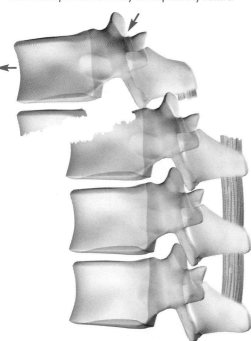

Pelvis—Introduction

Fractures of the pelvis can be complicated by injuries to the soft-tissues, including the urethra, bladder, bowel, nerves and vessels. As well as hemorrhage due to bony injury, vascular injuries may cause massive hemorrhage.

A normal pelvis is illustrated in Figure 10.

The mechanism of injury can be divided into:
1. AP compression (Figure 11)
2. lateral compression (Figures 12a and 12b)
3. vertical shear (Figure 13)

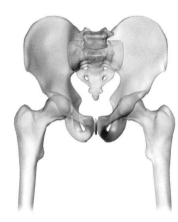

Figure 10. Normal pelvis.

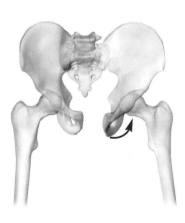

Figure 11. AP compression—lateral rotation of the fracture 'fragment'.

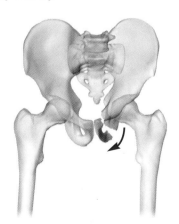

Figure 12a. Lateral compression— 'ring' or buckling.

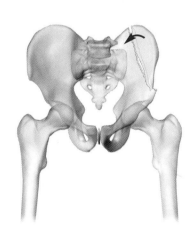

Figure 12b. Lateral compression—break.

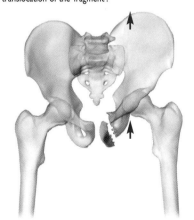

Figure 13. Vertical shear—disruption with superior translocation of the 'fragment'.

Pelvic views
• AP pelvis

Film-viewing routine
AP view
Look for:
• soft-tissue swelling within the pelvis, which may be due to hemorrhage

Look at:
• the cortex of the sacrum, iliac wings, ischium, acetabulum and pubic rami for a fracture
• the sacroiliac joints for disruption (as this is associated with a pelvic fracture) and the sacral arcuate lines for disruption
• the femur for a fracture

Figure 14. Stable fractures.

a) Avulsion fractures.

b) Isolated iliac wing fracture.

c) Unilateral fractures of the pubic rami.

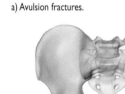
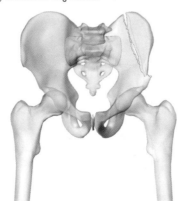
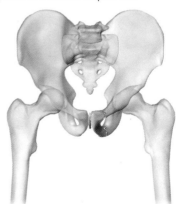

Figure 15. Unstable fractures.

a) Sacral fractures either in isolation or combined.

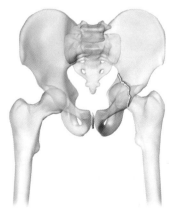

b) Posterior acetabular fractures +/- posterior dislocation.

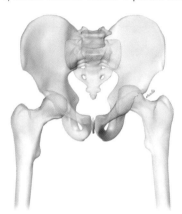

c) Acetabular roof fractures +/- central dislocation.

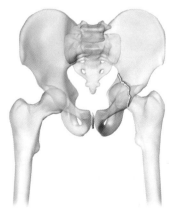

d) Symphysis pubis separation.

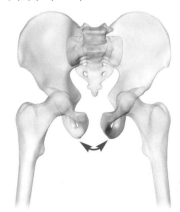

e) Hemipelvis ring fractures in two or more places.

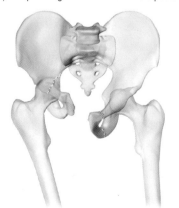

Additional information: stable and unstable fractures

The pelvis is a ring structure consisting of a posterior arch (sacrum and iliac wings extending to the acetabulum) and an anterior arch (extending anteriorly and inferiorly from the acetabulum). The pelvic 'ring' is like a pretzel; it rarely breaks in one place alone. Features associated with stable and unstable fractures are outlined below:

- a single break in the pelvic ring, e.g. an isolated pubic ramus fracture is usually stable
- most stable pelvic fractures involve the anterior arch
- stable fractures may still have associated visceral injury, e.g. medial pubic rami fractures with urethral trauma
- unstable fractures are usually multiple fractures of both anterior and posterior arches

Stable and unstable pelvic fractures are shown in Figures 14 and 15, respectively.

Case Studies

Case 1

Clinical details

This patient sustained a hyperflexion injury when her car was shunted from behind.

Figure 1. AP cervical spine.

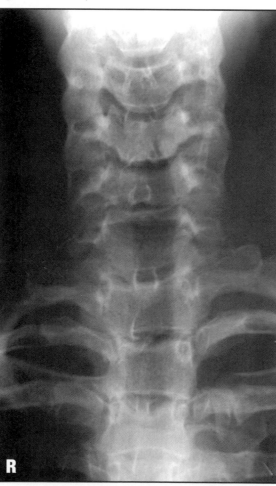

Figure 2. Lateral cervical spine.

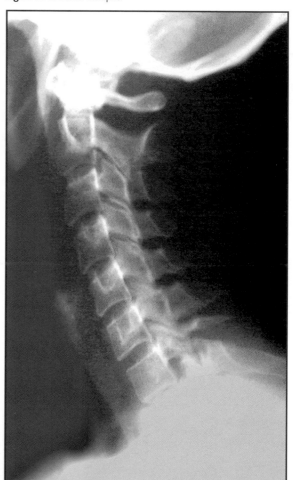

Radiological features

On the lateral view, there is a longitudinal fracture extending from the spinous process of C7, through the laminae and pedicles into the postero-lateral aspect of the C7 vertebral body. The ASL is interrupted by a step at C7/T1. On the AP view, when counting the spinous processes caudally, there appears to be an extra spinous process, which is a result of the spinous process fracture.

There is also widening of the interspinous distance as a result of both the spinous process fracture and disruption of the interspinous ligaments. The fracture line is visible on the AP view in the left C7 pedicle.

Diagnosis

Fracture of the posterior elements of C7 extending to the vertebral body.

Discussion

The widening of the interspinous distance is indicated on the AP and lateral views below (Figures 3 and 4, respectively). The ASL is outlined on Figure 4.

Figure 3. The AP view. The widening of the interspinous distance is indicated by arrows and the fracture of the left C7 pedicle is outlined.

Figure 4. The lateral view with the widening of the interspinous distance and the spinous process fracture indicated by a double-headed arrow. The ASL is also outlined showing the step at C7/T1.

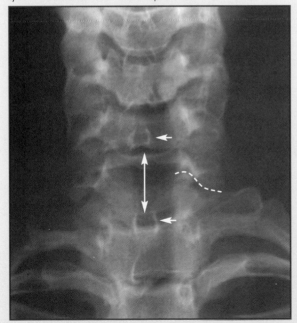

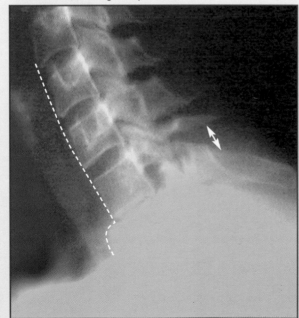

Case 2

Clinical details

This patient sustained a deceleration neck injury in a head-on-collision. His immediate films were deemed satisfactory. However, he re-presented 10 days later with tingling in his right hand in a C6 distribution. What radiological features are present?

Figure 1. Lateral cervical spine.

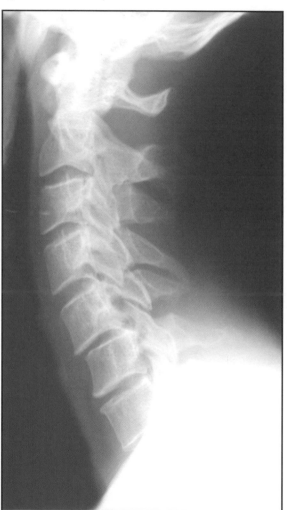

Figure 2. AP cervical spine.

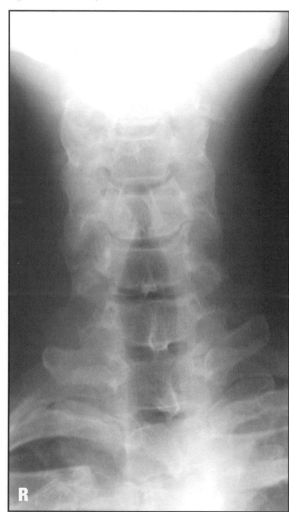

Radiological features

On the lateral view there is angulation at the C5/C6 intervertebral disc level, with loss of height of this disc space and anterior slip of C5 on C6. There is widening of the interspinous distance at the C5/C6 level on both the lateral and the AP views (implying posterior interspinous ligament disruption). On the lateral view, the facet joints are not aligned at the C5 level indicating a rotational subluxation of the facet joints (they are normally aligned above and below C5/C6). On the AP view, the spinous processes are not aligned at C5/C6.

Diagnosis

Unilateral facet joint dislocation at C5/C6.

Discussion

This is an unstable fracture. The features of this dislocation are outlined on the lateral and AP views (Figures 3 and 4, respectively).

Figure 3. The lateral view with the dislocation indicated by arrows. The angulation at the C5/C6 intervertebral disc level, with loss of height of this disc space and anterior slip of C5 on C6 is indicated by a single arrow head. The widening of the interspinous distance at its C5/C6 level is indicated by a double-headed arrow.

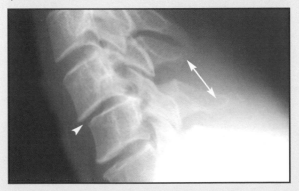

Figure 4. The AP view. The dashed line outlines that the spinous processes are not aligned at C5/C6.

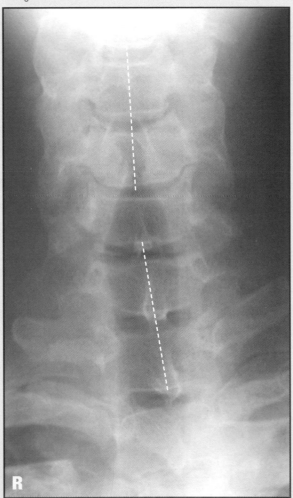

Case 3

Clinical details

This patient was digging in his back garden. Later in the day he had a sudden onset of pain in the lower cervical spine, which was worse on movement. What injury is present?

Figure 1. Lateral cervical spine.

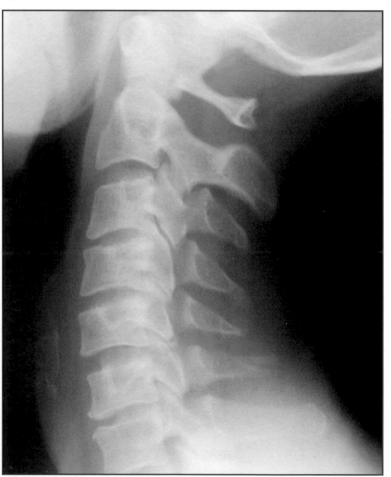

Radiological features

There is a fracture of the C6 spinous process, termed a 'clay shoveler's' fracture.

Diagnosis

C6 spinous process fracture (clay shoveler's fracture).

Discussion

This is an avulsion fracture of the spinous process due to a sudden load on a flexed spine. This is a stable fracture.

Case 4

Clinical details

This patient sustained a deceleration injury to their neck. What does the lateral film show?

Figure 1. Lateral cervical spine.

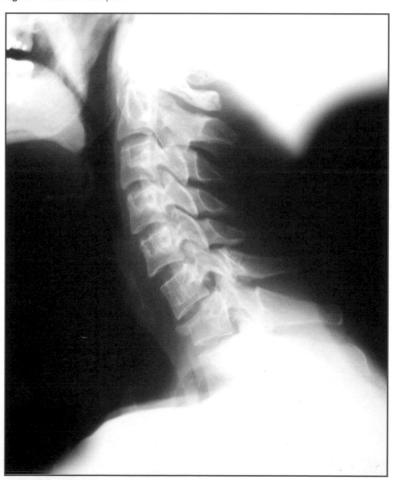

Radiological features

There is an anterior wedge fracture of the C7 vertebra with impaction of the superior end plate. The intervertebral disc height between C6 and C7 is narrowed and the C6 vertebra is subluxed anteriorly on the C7 vertebra (note the PSL is malaligned). In addition, the facet joints are perched, with the inferior articular facet of C6 sitting high on the superior articular facet of C7. There is widening of the interspinous distance implying separation of the interspinous ligaments.

Diagnosis

Hyperflexion injury with anterior wedge fracture of C7, and subluxation and perched facet joints at C6/C7. Spinous ligament rupture.

Case 5

Clinical details

This patient tripped, struck their jaw on the pavement and experienced sudden severe neck pain. The patient was brought to casualty in a rigid collar. What fracture is present from the lateral view?

Figure 1. Lateral cervical spine.

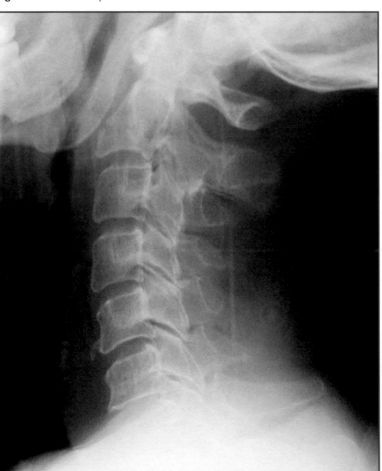

Radiological features

There is a fracture of the C2 vertebra extending from the body anteriorly through the pedicles and laminae almost to the spinous process. There is minor broadening of the pre-cervical soft-tissue at this level.

Diagnosis

Hyperextension injury with fracture of C2.

Discussion

This is an unstable fracture. The C2 fracture is outlined on the lateral view below (Figure 2).

Figure 2. The lateral cervical spine with the C2 fracture outlined.

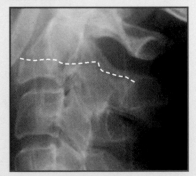

Case 6

Clinical details

This lady began to choke on a suspected fish bone and her grandson performed a vigorous Heimlich maneuver, which relieved the symptoms. However, the feeling of a foreign body in her throat recurred 20 minutes later. This film was taken 1 hour after the initial symptoms. What does it show?

Figure 1. Lateral cervical spine.

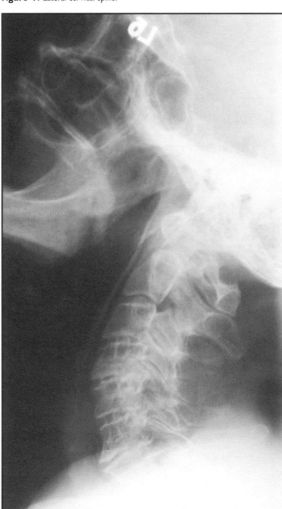

Radiological features

There is marked degenerate change in the cervical region of the spine and there is gas seen within the pre-cervical fascia.

Diagnosis

Pre-vertebral gas in the soft-tissue.

Discussion

The over vigorous coughing or Heimlich maneuver resulted in gas tracking up from a pneumo-mediastinum. The symptoms settled spontaneously. The region of gas is shown on the lateral view below (Figure 2).

Figure 2. Lateral cervical spine. The region of gas lies between the two sets of arrows.

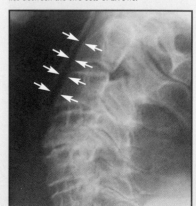

Case 7

Clinical details

This man tripped and fell at home.
What abnormalities can you see
on the initial film (Figure 1)?
What abnormalities can you see
on the subsequent film, taken
2 days later (Figure 2)?

Figure 1. Lateral cervical spine.

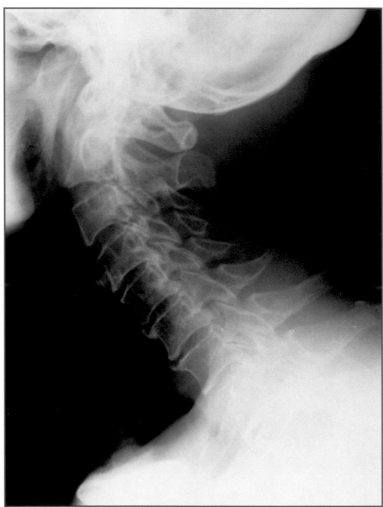

Radiological features

On the initial film, the PSL and SL are malaligned at C2/C3, being posteriorly displaced above C2/C3. There is increased intervertebral space anteriorly at C2/C3. However, no fracture line is seen. On the subsequent film a 'Hangman's' fracture is seen; a lucency between the body and posterior elements/pedicle of C2.

Diagnosis

Hangman's fracture of C2 (hyperflexion injury).

Discussion

This is an unstable fracture. Although the fracture itself cannot be seen on the initial films, the loss of alignment of two spinal lines and widened intervertebral space are a 'red flag', i.e. warning that this is an unstable spine.

Figure 2. Lateral cervical spine.

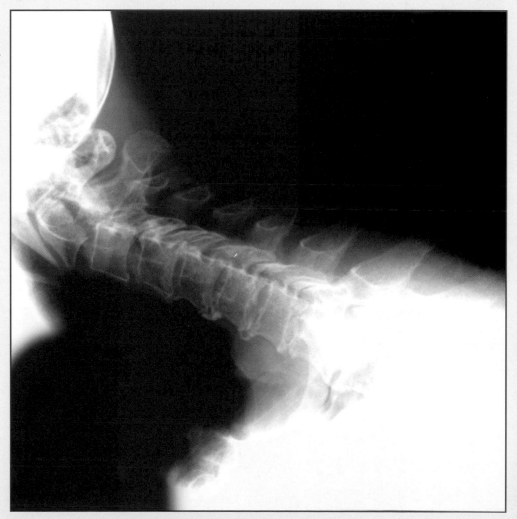

Case 8

Clinical details
This young man was involved in a road traffic accident (RTA). His car turned upside down and he hit his head on the roof.

Figure 1. Lateral cervical spine.

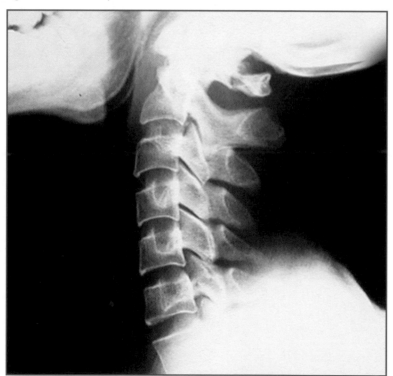

Figure 2. Lateral upper cervical spine (magnified view).

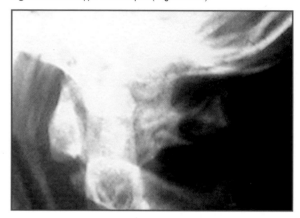

Figure 3. Peg view.

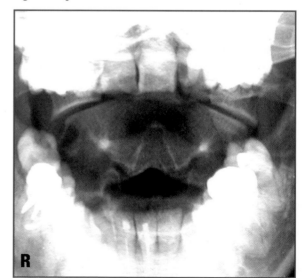

Radiological features

On the 'peg' view, the lateral masses of C1 lie lateral to the lateral masses of C2 (normally they are aligned, as illustrated in the *Rules and tools, Spine and axial skeleton*). On the lateral views, a fracture can be seen through the posterior elements of C1.

Diagnosis

Jefferson's fracture of C1.

Discussion

CT (not given) showed a fracture of the C1 ring at two sites, thus allowing the C1 lateral masses to move lateral to C2.

The fracture seen through the posterior elements of C1 is outlined on the lateral view below (Figure 4).

The dashed lines on the peg view (Figure 5) outline that the lateral masses of C1 lie lateral to the lateral masses of C2.

Figure 5. The peg view with position of the lateral masses indicated by dashed lines. The lateral masses of C1 are displaced laterally with respect to the lateral masses of C2.

Figure 4. The lateral view with the fracture outlined.

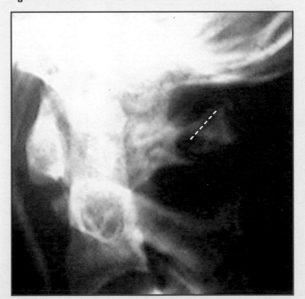

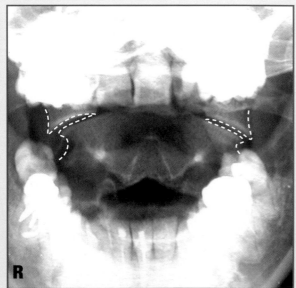

Case Studies

Case 9

Clinical details

This elderly patient fell at home and experienced a sudden onset of pain in the thoraco-lumbar region. What is the probable cause and is this stable?

Figure 1. Lateral thoracic spine.

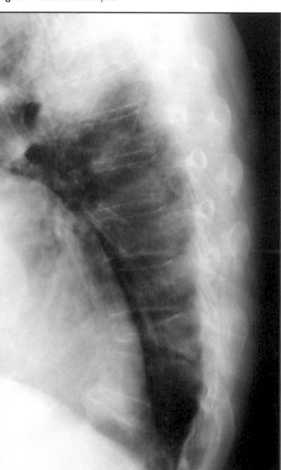

Figure 2. AP thoracic spine.

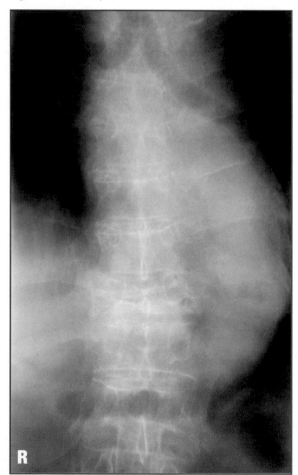

Radiological features

There is a stable wedge compression fracture of the T10 vertebra.

The loss of anterior height of the T10 vertebra is more pronounced than that of the posterior portion of the vertebral body.

Diagnosis

Vertebral wedge fracture of T10.

Discussion

This is a stable fracture. The wedge fracture of T10 is outlined on the lateral and AP views below (Figures 3 and 4, respectively).

Figure 3. The lateral view with the wedge fracture outlined.

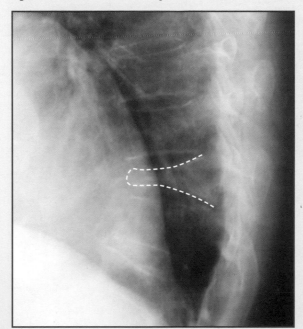

Figure 4. The AP view with the wedge fracture outlined.

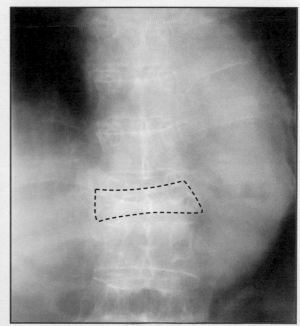

Case 10

Case 10

Clinical details

This child was sitting on the central rear seat when their car was shunted from behind. He complained of lower back pain.

(Radiographs courtesy of Dr K McHugh)

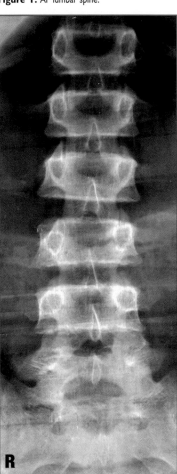

Figure 1. AP lumbar spine.

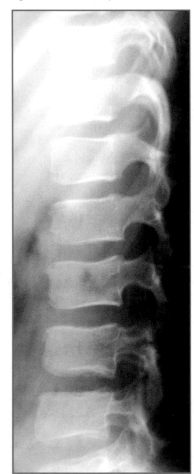

Figure 2. Lateral lumbar spine.

Radiological features

There is a longitudinal fracture seen extending from the L3 spinous process into the lamina, left transverse process and left pedicle. There is also a right transverse process fracture of L2 and L3.

Diagnosis

Chance fracture of L3 (hyperflexion injury) and right transverse process fracture of L2 and L3.

Discussion

The child was wearing the central rear lap belt causing a hyperflexion injury of the lumbar spine. This may be associated with abdominal trauma.

The longitudinal lucency on L3 is outlined on the AP and lateral views below (Figures 3 and 4, respectively). The right transverse process fractures are also indicated on Figure 3.

Figure 3. The AP view with a dashed line above and below the longitudinal lucency of L3 (chance fracture) and the right transverse process fractures indicated by arrows.

Figure 4. The lateral view with the L3 chance fracture outlined (through the L3 spinous process to the lamina).

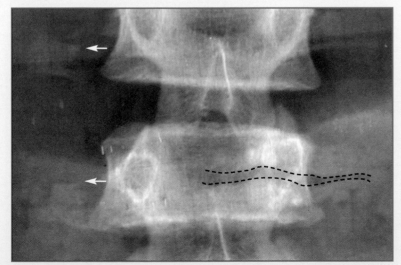

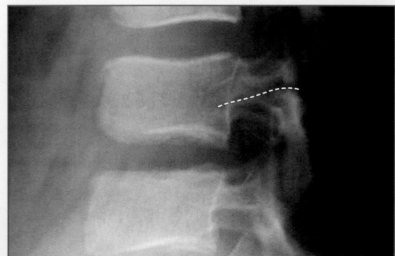

Case 11

Clinical details

This young active patient complained of longstanding lumbar pain.

Figure 1. Lateral lumbar spine.

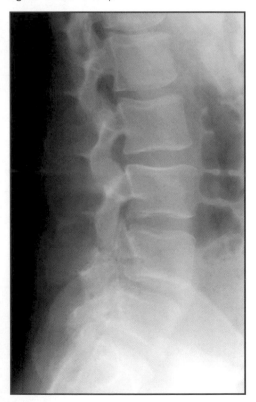

Radiological features

There are bilateral pars defects seen at the L4 level, with no resultant spondylolisthesis.

These pars defects are seen as a discontinuity (lucent line) in the pars interarticularis (part of the vertebral neural arch between the pedicle and the lamina).

Diagnosis

Bilateral L4 pars defect.

Discussion

Anterior subluxation of the vertebra above the defect may occur.

This abnormality is a relatively common cause of prolonged lower back pain in young adults.

The lucent line is outlined on the lateral view below (Figure 2).

Figure 2. The lateral view with the lucent line outlined.

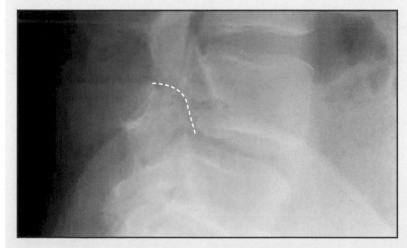

Case 12

Clinical details
This patient was driving a small car and shunted the vehicle in front. He sustained severe right hip pain.

Figure 1. Frontal pelvis.

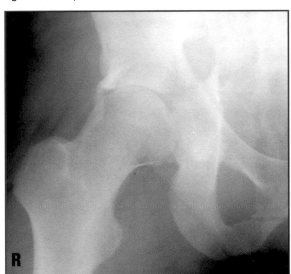

Figure 2. Axial CT scan.

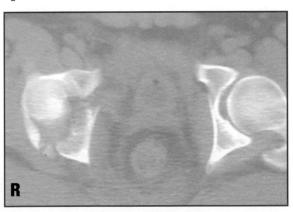

Radiological features
There is medial migration of the right femoral head with fractures of the medial and posterior acetabular walls evident on the frontal view. This is illustrated on the axial CT image.

Diagnosis
Unstable right acetabular fracture with medial migration of right femoral head.

Case 13

Clinical details

This patient was involved in a high velocity RTA and suffered extensive injuries including fractures of both femurs and ankles. This radiograph was taken after a laparotomy for extensive mesenteric hemorrhage. What fractures are present?

Figure 1. Frontal pelvis.

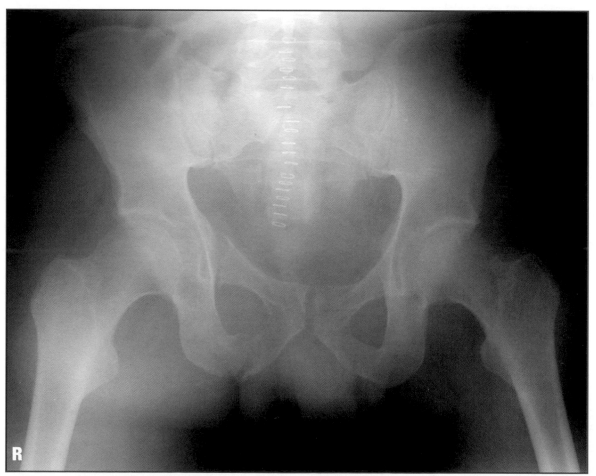

Radiological features

There is a fracture through the medial aspect of the right hemisacrum with a horizontally orientated fracture in the left hemisacrum. In addition there are fractures of the superior and inferior pubic rami on the right and a fracture through the superior pubic ramus/symphysis pubis on the left. Surgical clips are present in the midline from closure of the laparotomy.

Diagnosis

Complex unstable pelvic fracture.

Discussion

The reconstructed axial CT shows the same fractures in 2D (Figure 2).

The injuries are indicated by arrows on the frontal view below (Figure 3).

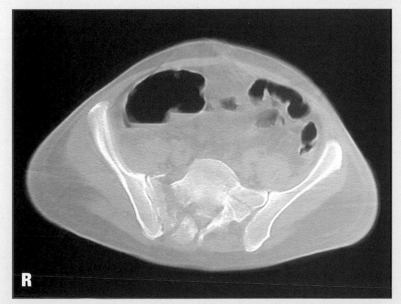

Figure 2. Axial CT pelvis.

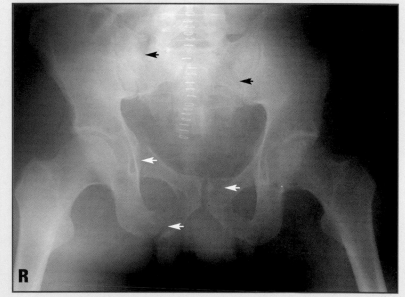

Figure 3. The frontal view with the complex pelvic fracture indicated by arrows.

Case 14

Clinical details

This elderly man was knocked to the ground whilst shopping. He was able to stand, although he had great discomfort in his right groin.

Radiological features

There are unilateral right-sided fractures of the superior and inferior pubic rami.

Diagnosis

Right superior and inferior pubic rami fractures.

Discussion

The following fractures are possible causes of groin or hip pain in elderly patients after trauma:

1. fracture of the neck of the femur
2. pubic rami fractures

The fractures are indicated on the frontal view below.

Figure 1. Frontal pelvis.

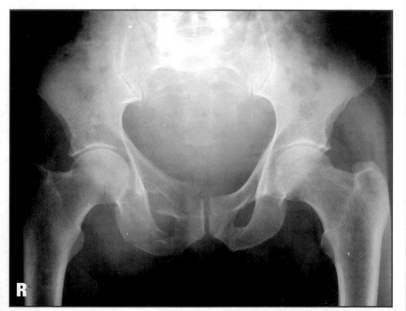

Figure 2. The frontal pelvis with fractures indicated by arrows.

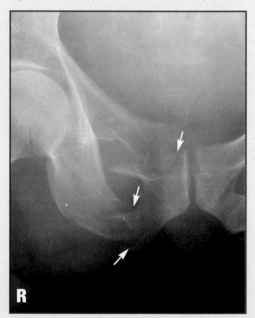

Upper Limb

Rules and Tools

Introduction

Fractures of the upper limb are very common, particularly around the wrist. They are often found in elderly patients.

It is important to evaluate and X-ray the joint above and below the fracture as there may be a dislocation or a second fracture. This does not usually apply to a simple Colles' fracture of the distal radius and ulna styloid.

Shoulder

Shoulder views
- Anteroposterior (AP)
- 'Y' view
- Axial view

Film-viewing routine

AP view (Figures 1a and 1b)
Check:
- alignment of the glenoid and humerus (see line 1, Figure 1a)
- alignment of the acromion and clavicle (see line 2, Figure 1a)

Look at:
- the cortical edge of the humerus, clavicle and ribs for fractures
- the chest (if fractures have been found), to make sure there is no accompanying pneumothorax

'Y' view (Figures 2a and 2b)
Check:
- the humeral head overlies the 'Y' shape made by the body of the scapula, the coracoid (anterior) and the acromion (posterior); if it does not, then there is a gleno-humeral dislocation (anteriorly or posteriorly)

Axial view (Figures 3a and 3b)
First:
- orientate the film by identifying the acromion (posterior) and the coracoid process (anterior)

Check:
- the glenoid and humeral head are aligned (see line 1, Figure 3a)

Figure 1a. AP view of the shoulder.

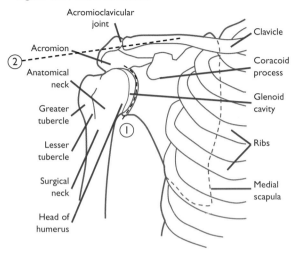

Acromioclavicular joint

Acromion

②

Anatomical neck

Greater tubercle

Lesser tubercle

Surgical neck

Head of humerus

Clavicle

Coracoid process

Glenoid cavity

Ribs

Medial scapula

①

Figure 2a. 'Y' view of the shoulder.

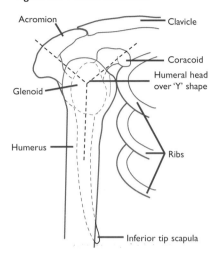

Acromion

Glenoid

Humerus

Clavicle

Coracoid

Humeral head over 'Y' shape

Ribs

Inferior tip scapula

Figure 3a. Axial view of the shoulder.

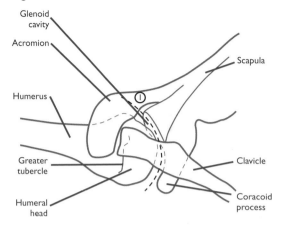

Glenoid cavity

Acromion

Humerus

Greater tubercle

Humeral head

Scapula

Clavicle

Coracoid process

①

Figure 1b. Normal AP radiograph of the shoulder.

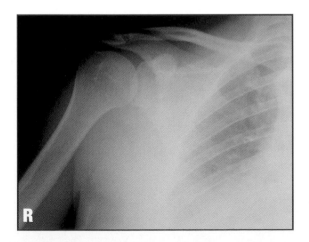

Figure 2b. Normal 'Y' radiograph of the shoulder.

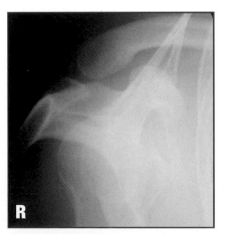

Figure 3b. Normal axial radiograph of the shoulder.

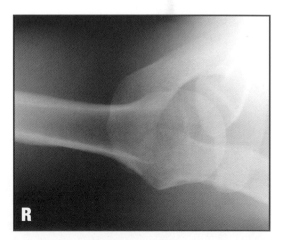

Elbow

Elbow views
• AP
• Lateral

Film-viewing routine
AP and lateral views (Figures 4a/b and 5a/b, respectively)
Check:
• a straight line can be drawn through both the radius and capitellum in all positions; (see line 1, Figures 4a and 5a); if not, a radial head dislocation may be present

Lateral view (Figures 5a and 5b)
Look for:
• a raised anterior (most common) or posterior fat pad—this is caused by a joint effusion raising the pad of fat that is normally closely applied to the joint (illustrated in Figure 5a)

Check:
• a line drawn down the anterior humeral cortex passes through the middle third of the capitellum (see line 2, Figure 5a); if these structures are not in line, there may be a supracondylar fracture of the humerus

Look at:
• the cortex of the radial head— run your eye around it to look for a subtle fracture (this is the commonest elbow fracture). Failure to identify a fracture here does not exclude one in the presence of an effusion

Figure 4a. AP view of the elbow.

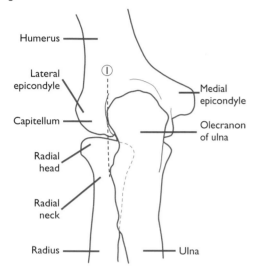

Humerus

Lateral
epicondyle

Capitellum

Radial
head

Radial
neck

Radius

①

Medial
epicondyle

Olecranon
of ulna

Ulna

Figure 4b. Normal AP radiograph of the elbow.

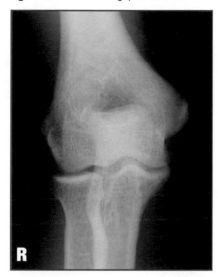

Figure 5a. Lateral view of the elbow.

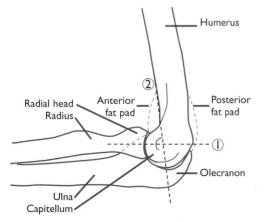

Radial head
Radius

Anterior
fat pad

②

Humerus

Posterior
fat pad

①

Olecranon

Ulna

Capitellum

Figure 5b. Normal lateral radiograph of the elbow.

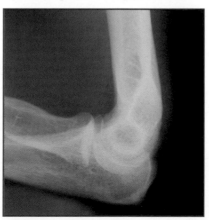

Wrist and hand

Wrist and hand views
- AP
- Lateral
- Dedicated scaphoid views

Film-viewing routine

AP view (Figures 6a and 6b)
Look at:
- the cortex of the distal radius and ulna for a fracture
- the distal radius for a dense sclerotic band, indicating an impacted fracture
- the two rows of carpal bones—a line drawn along the top and bottom of the carpal bones in each row should be continuous without any steps (as shown by lines 1, 2 and 3 in Figure 6a); if not this suggests a carpal dislocation
- the spaces between each of the carpal bones, which should be roughly parallel; this is lost in carpal dislocation
- the shape of the lunate, which should be rectangular on the AP view; if not, suspect a lunate or peri-lunate dislocation (check the radio-capitate-lunate alignment on the lateral view)

Lateral view (Figures 7a and 7b)
Check:
- the cortex of the distal radius and ulna, including the styloid process to see if it is intact and if there is any angulation
- a line can be drawn through the radius, lunate and capitate (see line 1, Figures 7a and 7b)—if not suspect a lunate or peri-lunate dislocation

Additional information
The USA and UK nomenclature for some carpal bones differ:
- the scaphoid (UK), is known as the navicular (US)
- the triquetral (UK), is known as the triangular (US)
- the trapezium (UK), is known as the greater multangular (US)
- the trapezoid (UK), is known as the lesser multangular (US)

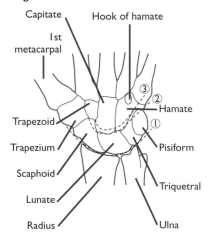

Figure 6a. AP view of the wrist.

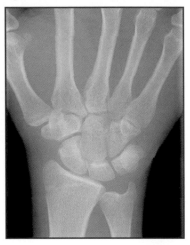

Figure 6b. Normal AP radiograph of the wrist.

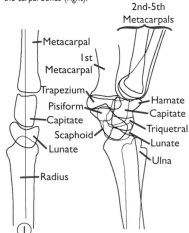

Figure 7a. Lateral view of the wrist showing the radius, capitate and lunate (left) and all of the carpal bones (right).

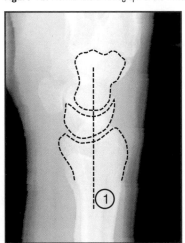

Figure 7b. Normal lateral radiograph of the wrist.

Pediatric fractures

Children have different injuries to adults due to their bone structure (which is softer) and their unfused epiphyses.

When a force is applied to an unfused bone it may:
• bend without a cortical break—bowing
• develop a cortical 'wrinkle'—torus fracture
• develop a cortical break on one side—greenstick fracture

Figure 8 illustrates these pediatric fractures.

Figure 8. Normal anatomy of unfused bone and sub-types of pediatric metaphyseal fractures.

a) Normal

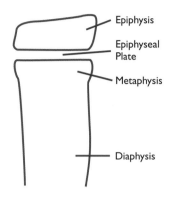

Epiphysis

Epiphyseal Plate

Metaphysis

Diaphysis

b) Bowing

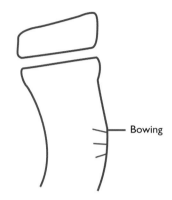

Bowing

c) Torus fracture

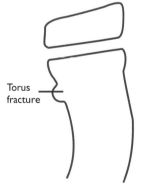

Torus fracture

d) Greenstick fracture

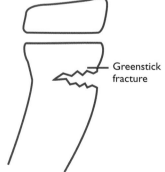

Greenstick fracture

Additional information

- A fracture line that crosses the epiphyseal plate can impair future epiphyseal growth
- Epiphyseal fractures are subdivided according to the Salter–Harris classification (Figure 9, a useful mnemonic for remembering the five sub-types is shown in the left-hand column)
- The mnemonic CRITOL lists the order in which the epiphyses of the elbow ossify and become visible on plain radiographs (Table 1). This is important to remember in order not to misdiagnose normally sited epiphyses as fractures, and not to overlook a dislocated epiphysis

Figure 9. Salter–Harris fractures involving epiphyseal growth centers.

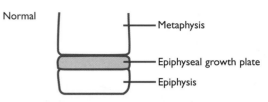

Mnemonic	Type	Illustration	Comments
S Separation	I		
A Above (i.e. metaphysis)	II		Most common
L Lower (i.e. epiphysis)	III		
T Through (i.e. epiphysis and metaphysis)	IV		
(E) R Rammed	V		Worst prognosis

Table 1. The mnemonic CRITOL of the appearance of epiphyses of the elbow.

Epiphysis	Abbreviation	Approximate age of ossification and appearance on X-ray (years)
Capitellum	C	1
Radial head	R	5
Inner (i.e. medial) epicondyle	I	5
Trochlea	T	10
Olecranon	O	10
Lateral epicondyle	L	10–11

Case Studies

Case 1

Clinical details

This patient arrived at the Emergency Department in a lot of pain holding his left arm following a fall.

Figure 1. AP shoulder.

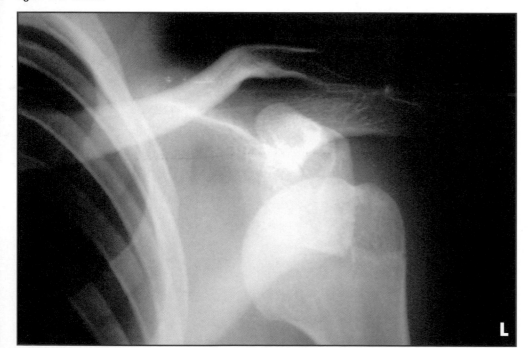

Figure 2. 'Y' shoulder.

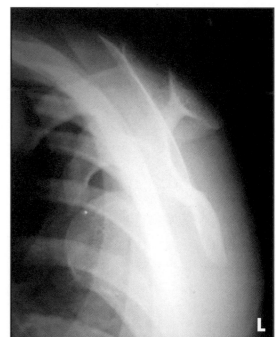

Radiological features

On a normal AP view of the shoulder, the glenoid and humeral head should parallel each other. In this patient the humeral head lies anterior and inferior to the glenoid on both the 'Y' and AP views. Therefore this is an anterior dislocation of the shoulder.

Diagnosis

Anterior dislocation of shoulder.

Discussion

The 'Y' view position was easier for the patient, as it involved less movement. The 'Y' is formed from the junction of the scapular blade inferiorly, the acromion (posteriorly) and the coracoid (anteriorly). The humeral head should overlie the 'Y' and if it does not there is a dislocation. The 'Y shape' is outlined on the 'Y' view opposite (Figure 3).

Figure 3. The 'Y' view with the 'Y shape' outlined.

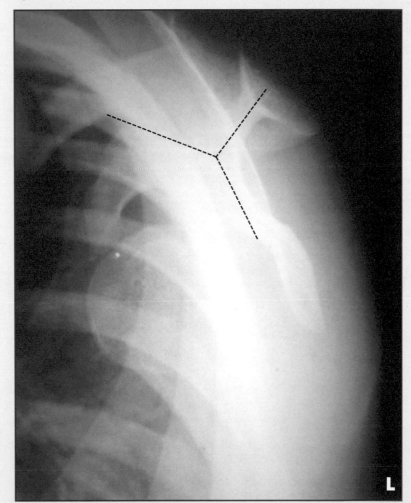

Case 2

Clinical details

The casualty officer suspected an anterior dislocation of the shoulder in this patient and accordingly reduced the shoulder; do the pre-and post-reduction views confirm his suspicion?

Figure 1. Pre-reduction AP shoulder.

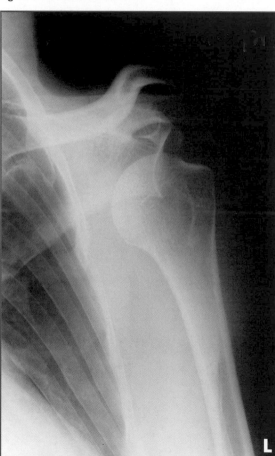

Figure 2. Post-reduction AP shoulder.

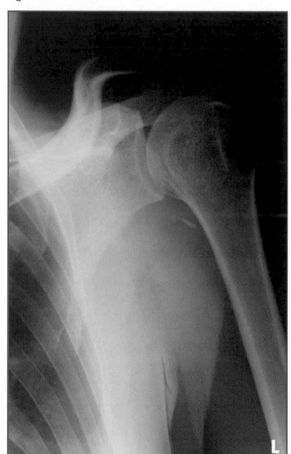

Figure 3. Pre-reduction 'Y' shoulder.

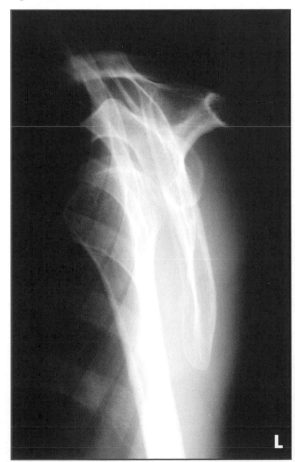

Figure 4. Post-reduction 'Y' shoulder.

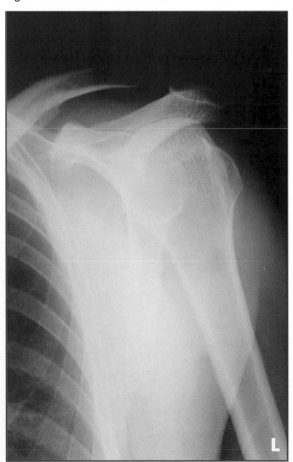

Radiological features

Yes, the pre- and post-reduction views do confirm this. The pre-reduction AP and 'Y' views demonstrate that the humeral head lies anterior and inferior to the glenoid. After reduction (note the 'Y' view is not perfectly positioned), the humeral head once again lies within the glenoid.

Diagnosis

Anterior shoulder dislocation.

Case 3

Clinical details
Anterior shoulder dislocation was
suspected in this patient.

Figure 1. Pre-reduction AP shoulder.

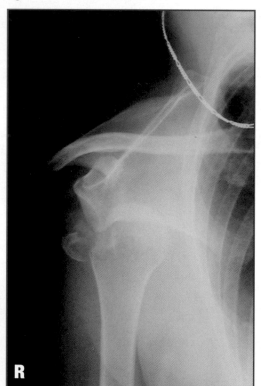

Figure 2. Pre-reduction 'Y' shoulder.

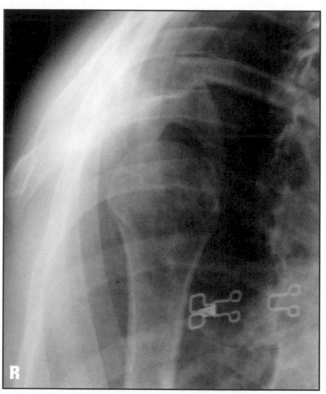

Radiological features

There is an anterior dislocation of the humeral head, but there is also a fracture of the greater tuberosity.

Diagnosis

Anterior shoulder dislocation and fracture of the greater tuberosity.

Discussion

In 15% of cases, an anterior dislocation is accompanied by a fracture of the greater tuberosity. This is not the same as a Hill-Sachs defect, which is a depression fracture of the posterolateral surface of the humeral head as a result of its impact against the glenoid rim.

The fracture of the greater tuberosity is indicated on the pre-reduction AP view opposite (Figure 3).

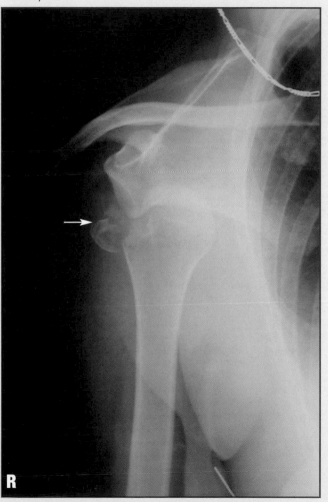

Figure 3. The pre-reduction AP view with the fracture of the greater tuberiosity indicated by an arrow.

Case 4

Clinical details

This man fell whilst playing basketball. These X-rays were requested to exclude glenohumeral dislocation.

Figure 1. AP shoulder.

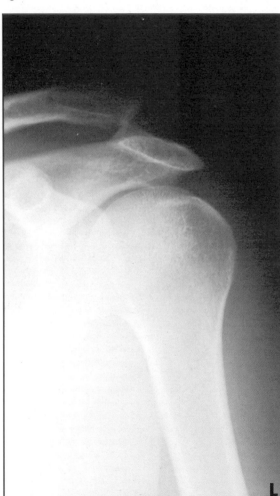

Figure 2. 'Y' shoulder.

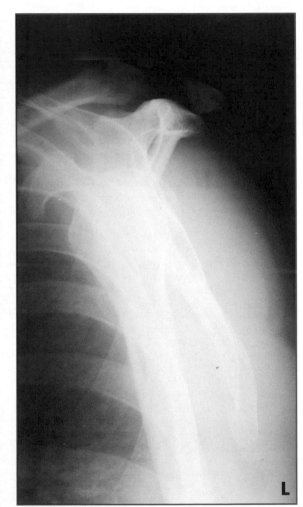

Radiological features

There is no glenohumeral dislocation. On the 'Y' view, the humeral head overlies the center of the 'Y' and so is normal. However, the acromion and clavicle are not aligned. Usually a line can be drawn between the inferior surface of the acromion and clavicle, but in this case the clavicle is raised in relation to the acromion. Loss of alignment has resulted due to injury of the coracoclavicular ligament. Weight-bearing views accentuate the acromioclavicular (AC) joint space and are helpful if there is doubt with the non-weight-bearing views.

Diagnosis

Left AC joint dislocation (grade III coracoclavicular injury).

Discussion

Injuries to the coracoclavicular ligament are classified into the following three categories: sprain (grade I), subluxation (grade II) and dislocation (grade III). Grade III injuries can be seen on a plain film but weight-bearing views may be needed for grade II. Mild widening of the AC joint space may be observed on the non-weight-bearing view with a grade I injury, but nothing else.

Figure 3 is a more obvious example of a grade III AC dislocation.

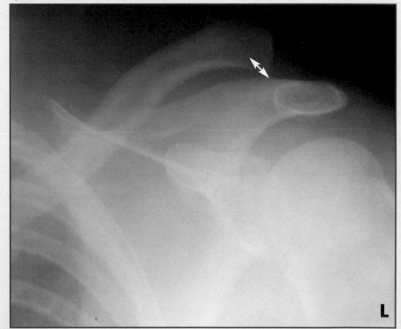

Figure 3. An AP shoulder with a more obvious grade III AC dislocation indicated by a double-headed arrow.

Case 5

What radiological feature is present
in this patient?

Radiological features
There is a fracture of the surgical
neck of the humerus, which is best
seen on the externally rotated view.

Diagnosis
Fracture of surgical neck of
humerus.

Discussion
The humeral head is not dislocated
on the 'Y' view although it is
displaced inferiorly probably due to
a joint effusion.

Figure 1. AP shoulder.

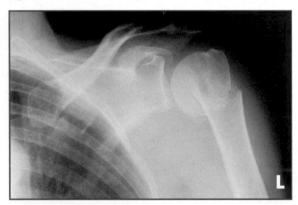

Figure 2. AP externally rotated shoulder.

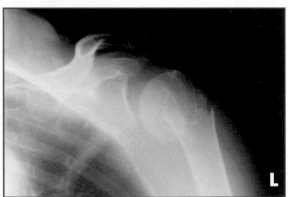

Figure 3. 'Y' shoulder.

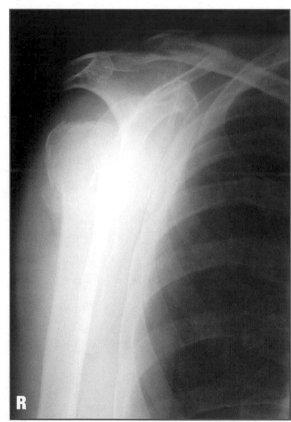

Case 6

Clinical details

This lady presented with shortness of breath and the casualty officer diagnosed left ventricular failure on the basis of a large heart, peri-hilar haziness and interstitial lines. What other incidental finding did she notice on the chest X-ray (CXR)?

Figure 1. CXR.

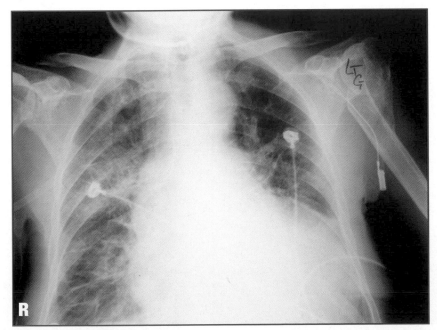

Radiological features

There is an old fracture of the neck of the left humerus (partly hidden by the side marker) with no union.

Diagnosis

Left ventricular failure and fracture of the neck of the left humerus.

Case Studies

Case 7

Is there any abnormality of
the shoulder?

Diagnosis
Normal. No fracture or dislocation.

Figure 1. AP shoulder.

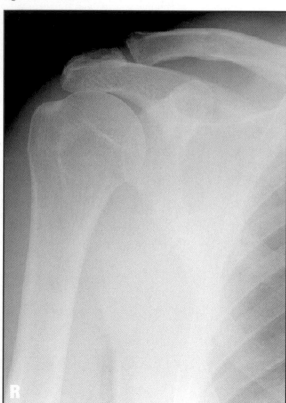

Figure 2. 'Y' shoulder.

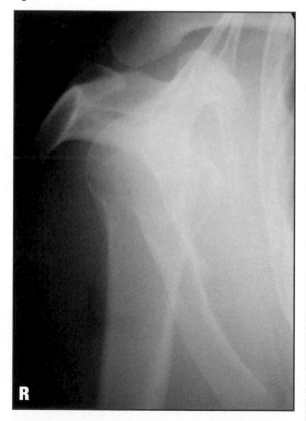

Case 8

Clinical details
This patient presented with pain
in her forearm but was unable
to localize the pain further.

Figure 1. AP wrist.

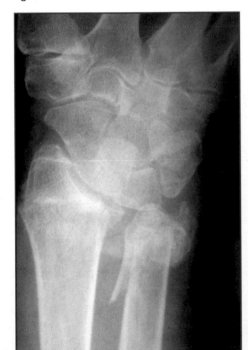

Figure 2. Lateral wrist.

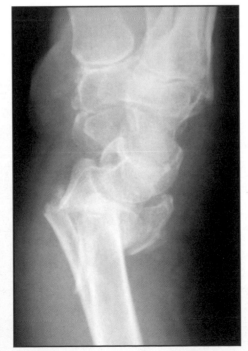

Radiological features
There is a fracture of the distal
radius, which involves the articular
surface—a break in the cortex
is visible on the dorsal part of
the radius. The distal fragment
is not angulated.

Diagnosis
Fracture of distal radius.

Discussion
If the distal fragment were
angulated, the fracture would
be classified according to the
angulation as follows:
1. Dorsal angulation—Barton's
   fracture
2. Volar angulation—reverse
   Barton's fracture

Case 9

Clinical details

This young man fell and twisted his arm.

Figure 1. AP elbow and shoulder.

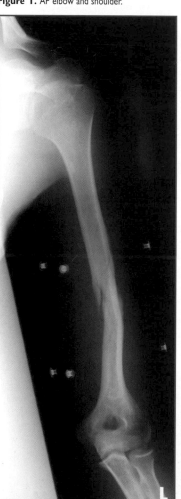

Figure 2. Lateral elbow and shoulder.

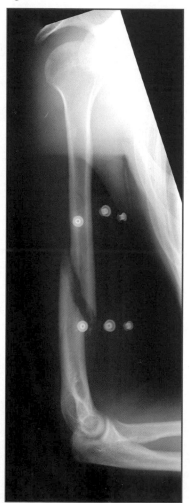

Radiological features

There is an obvious, displaced spiral fracture of the humerus.

Diagnosis

Left spiral fracture of humerus.

Discussion

The radial nerve runs around the humeral shaft and so in such cases it is important to assess whether its function has been affected by the fracture.

Case 10

Clinical details
This lady fell onto her elbow.

Figure 1. Lateral elbow.

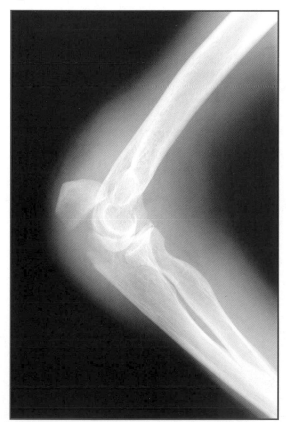

Radiological features
There is soft-tissue swelling, but no raised fat pads. There is a fracture of the olecranon, which is displaced.

Diagnosis
Olecranon fracture.

Discussion
The fracture was subsequently fixed with wires and pins, as shown on the lateral radiograph below (Figure 2).

Figure 2. Fracture fixed with wires and pins (lateral elbow).

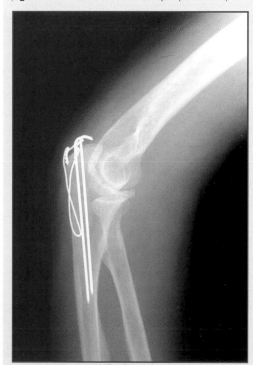

Case 11

What is the abnormality in this patient?

Radiological features

There is a fracture of the radial head on the AP view of the elbow. Raised anterior and posterior fat pads are visible.

Diagnosis

Radial head fracture.

Figure 1. AP elbow.

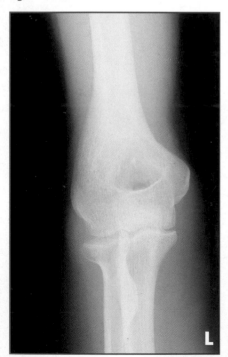

Figure 2. Lateral elbow.

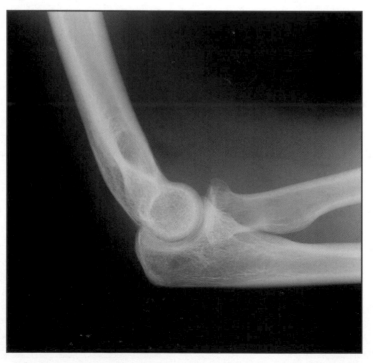

Case 12

Clinical details

Is this elbow fracture of a 12-year-old girl the most common type in an unfused skeleton?

Diagnosis

Fracture of radial neck.

Discussion

This is not the most common type of elbow fracture in an unfused skeleton. In children, particularly those under 10 years old, supracondylar fractures are most common. The fracture is indicated on the AP view (Figure 3).

Figure 1. AP elbow.

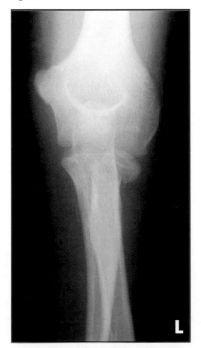

Figure 2. Lateral elbow.

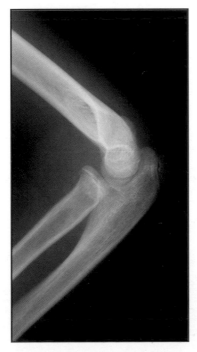

Figure 3. The AP view with the fracture indicated by an arrow.

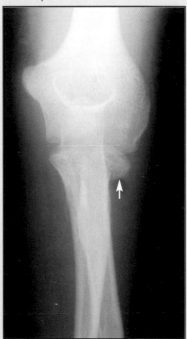

Case 13

Clinical details

This 50-year-old man fell onto his outstretched hand. What injury has he sustained? Is there any soft-tissue evidence of a fracture?

Figure 1. Lateral elbow.

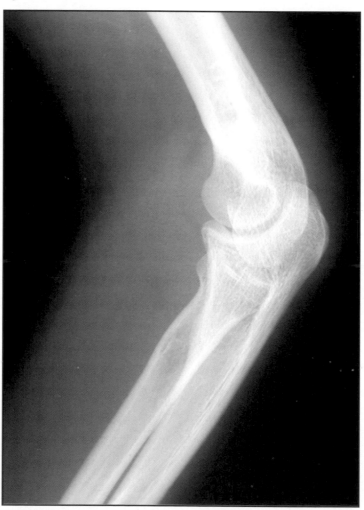

Radiological features

Raised anterior and posterior fat pads mean that there is a definite intraarticular fracture. There is in fact a fracture of the radial head.

Diagnosis

Radial head fracture.

Discussion

This is the most common elbow injury in an adult. On the lateral view opposite, the raised fat pads and fracture are indicated (Figure 2).

If the fracture line is not seen initially, raised fat pads (due to an elbow effusion) warrant immobilization and an X-ray should be taken again in 10 days time. Figure 3 shows a more obvious fracture of the radial head on a lateral view.

Figure 2. The lateral view with the raised fat pads outlined and the fracture indicated by an arrow.

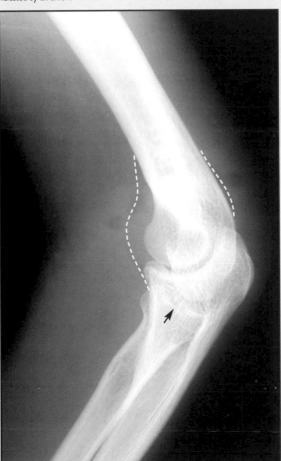

Figure 3. Lateral elbow with an obvious radial head fracture visible.

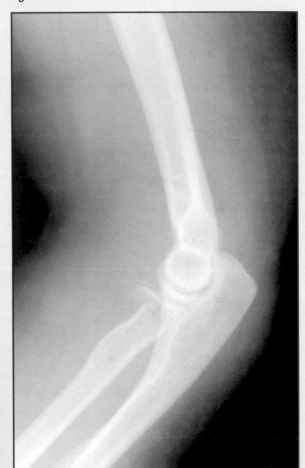

Case 14

What is the abnormality
in this patient?

Figure 1. AP elbow.

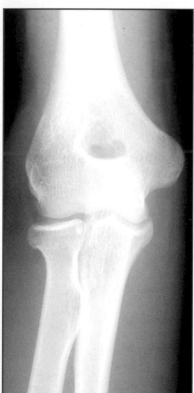

Figure 2. Lateral elbow.

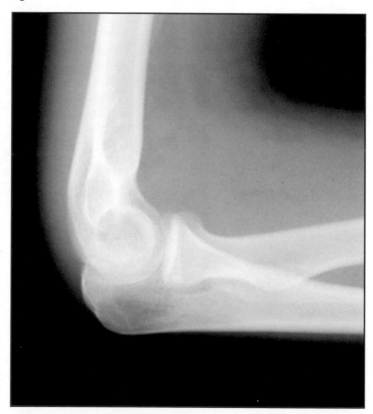

Radiological features

There is a fracture of the radial head on the AP view of the elbow. It can be very hard to identify a fracture on the lateral view, once again illustrating the importance of two views. If a fracture line cannot be seen, look for an effusion. A raised anterior fat pad is visible.

Diagnosis

Radial head fracture.

Discussion

A radial head fracture is the most common elbow fracture in an adult (a supracondylar fracture is the most common elbow fracture in a child).

Normally the anterior and posterior fat pads are closely applied to the joint. If there is an elbow effusion, e.g. the joint fills with blood after trauma, the fat pads are lifted by the effusion. In such a case, the posterior fat pad becomes visible, and the anterior fat pad, which normally can be seen as a small triangle, is lifted outward from the humerus in a sail shape. Raised fat pads are strongly suggestive of an intraarticular elbow fracture, but they may be absent in a fracture where the joint capsule is ruptured. If raised fat pads are observed but no fracture is seen, immobilize the elbow, X-ray again in 10 days time and re-assess for a fracture. The fracture and raised fat pad are indicated on the AP and lateral views below (Figures 3 and 4, respectively).

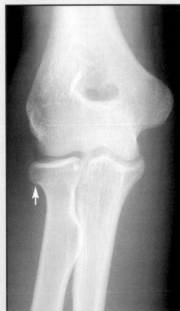

Figure 3. The AP view with the fracture indicated by an arrow.

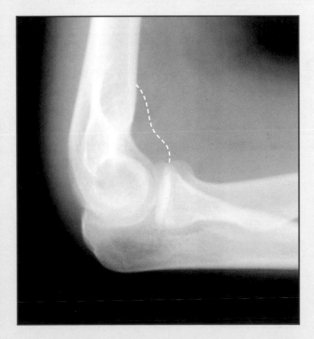

Figure 4. The lateral view with the raised anterior fat pad outlined.

Case 15

Is there a fracture here?

Figure 1. AP elbow.

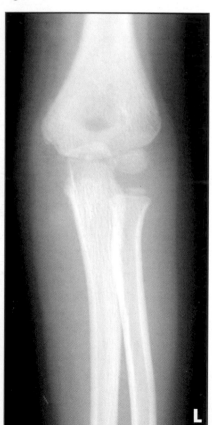

Figure 2. Lateral elbow.

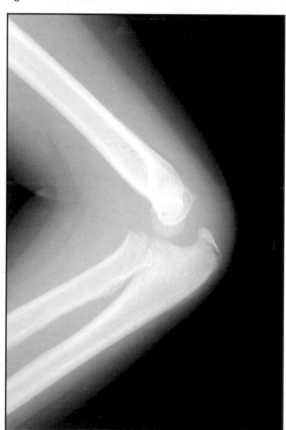

Radiological features

Yes, there is a fracture of the olecranon metaphysis, which is slightly displaced. This mimics the appearance of an olecranon epiphysis and therefore could be dismissed as normal.

Diagnosis

Fracture of olecranon metaphysis.

Discussion

In this child the medial epicondylar epiphysis is just visible, but not the trochlea. Therefore, the olecranon epiphysis should definitely not be seen and so the fragment must be a fracture (refer to the mnemonic CRITOL section in the *Rules and tools, Upper limb*). A film taken 3 weeks later shows callus formation confirming that there was a fracture (Figure 3).

Figure 3. Lateral elbow view taken 3 weeks later showing callus formation (indicated by an arrow).

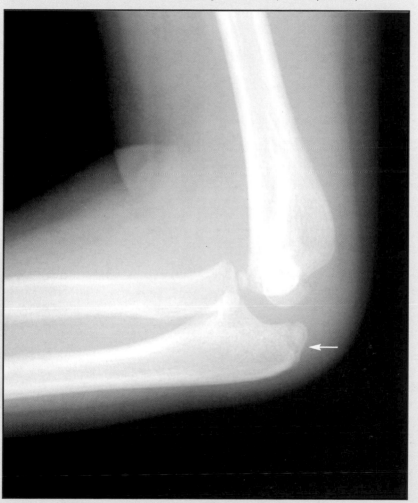

Case 16

Clinical details

This child refused to move his elbow after falling. What are the abnormalities?

Figure 1. AP elbow.

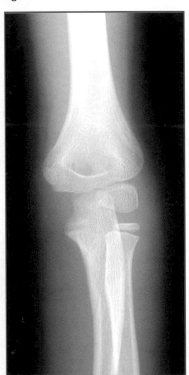

Figure 2. Lateral elbow.

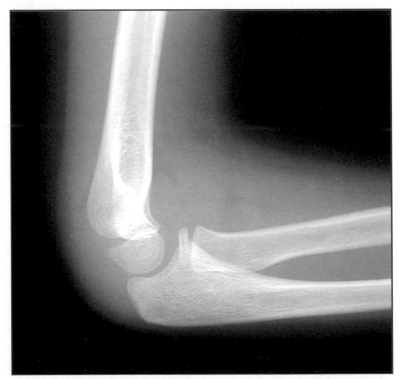

Radiological features

The following can be seen: raised posterior and anterior fat pads; no break in the cortex of the humerus; and normal radio-capitellar alignment. The presence of raised fat pads even without a cortical break strongly suggests a supracondylar fracture.

Diagnosis

Supracondylar fracture.

Discussion

The raised posterior and anterior fat pads are indicated on the lateral view opposite (Figure 3).

Figure 3. The lateral view with the raised anterior and posterior fat pads outlined.

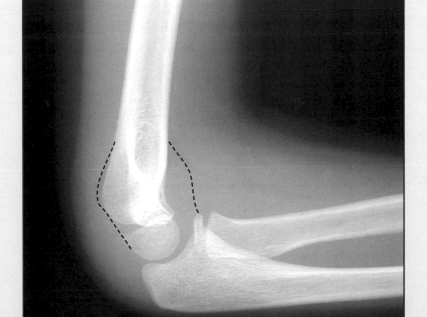

Case 17

Clinical details

This child fell and refused to move her arm. What are the abnormalities?

Figure 1. AP elbow.

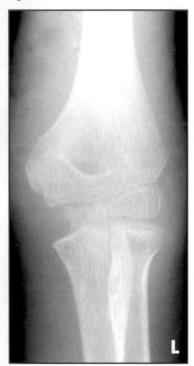

Figure 2. Lateral elbow.

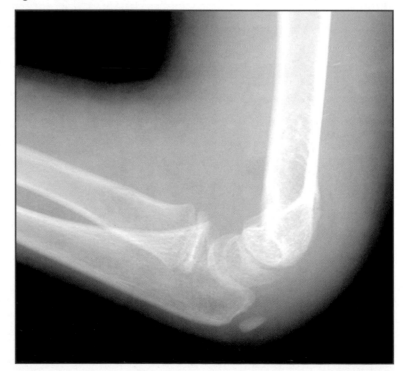

Radiological features

This child has a supracondylar fracture.

The fat pads are raised. On the lateral view, if a line is drawn along the anterior humerus, it bisects more than one-third of the capitellum and so the anterior humeral line alignment is disrupted. A break on the lateral aspect of the cortex is also visible on the AP view.

Diagnosis

Supracondylar fracture.

Discussion

The fracture is indicated on the AP view below (Figure 3). A line drawn along the anterior humerus is shown below on the lateral view (Figure 4).

Figure 4. The lateral view with the line drawn along the anterior humerus bisecting more than one-third of the capitellum. The raised fat pads are also outlined.

Figure 3. The AP view with the fracture indicated by arrows.

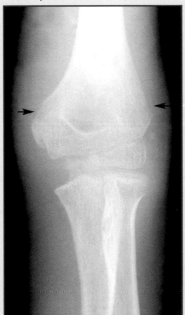

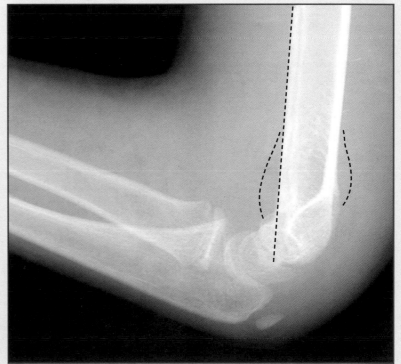

Case 18

Clinical details
This schoolgirl fell in
the playground.

Figure 1. AP wrist.

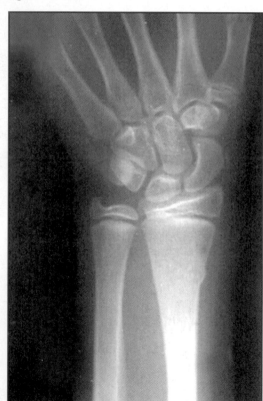

Figure 2. Lateral oblique wrist.

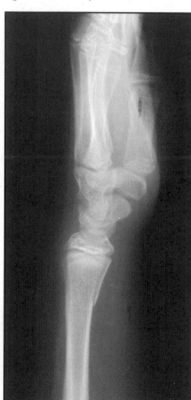

Figure 3. AP oblique wrist.

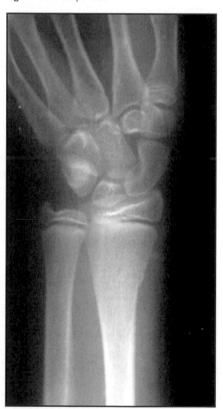

Radiological features

There is a torus fracture of the metadiaphysis (i.e. where the metaphysis and diaphysis meet) of the radius. There is slight volar angulation of the distal part of the radius.

Diagnosis

Torus fracture of metadiaphysis of radius.

Discussion

Both torus fractures and greenstick fractures can occur in children because their bones are relatively supple (see *Rules and tools, Upper limb*). The most common site is the metaphysis of the forearm.

A torus fracture is a slight buckling of the cortex, rather than an actual break in the cortex, with little or no angulation of the bone. A torus fracture is usually a consequence of a longitudinal compression force.

A greenstick fracture is a consequence of an angular force, resulting in a break of the cortex on one side of the bone with accompanied angulation.

The torus fracture is indicated on the AP and lateral oblique views opposite (Figures 4 and 5, respectively).

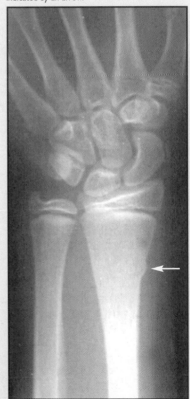

Figure 4. The AP view with the fracture indicated by an arrow.

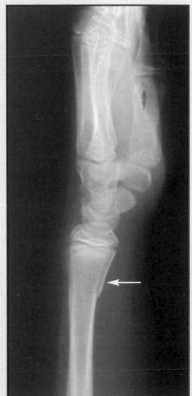

Figure 5. The lateral oblique view with the fracture indicated by an arrow.

Case 19

Clinical details
This boy fell over while
playing football.

Figure 1. AP wrist.

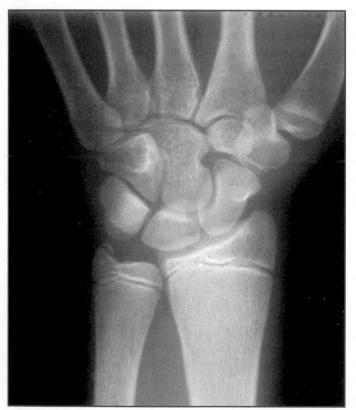

Figure 2. Lateral wrist.

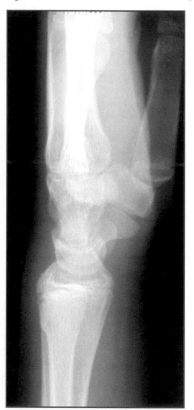

Figure 3. Oblique AP wrist.

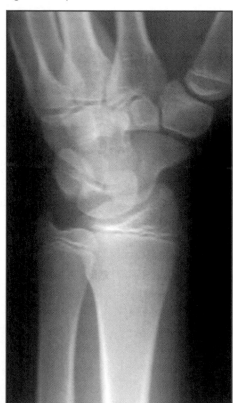

Radiological features

There is a fracture of the ulnar styloid. There is also a torus fracture of the radius, which can be observed on the lateral and oblique views by following the line of the metaphysis upwards.

Diagnosis

Ulnar styloid fracture and torus fracture of the radius.

Discussion

The ulnar styloid fracture is indicated on the AP view opposite (Figure 4).

The torus fracture is indicated on the lateral view opposite (Figure 5).

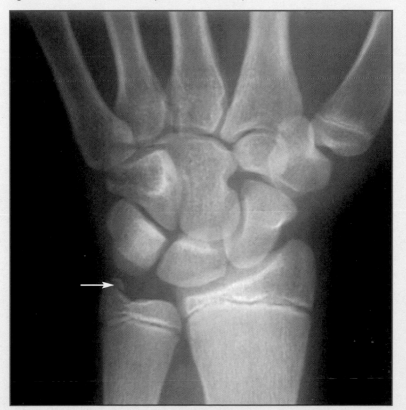

Figure 4. The AP view with the ulnar styloid fracture indicated by an arrow.

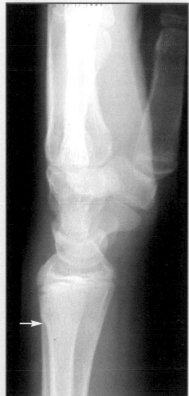

Figure 5. The lateral view with the torus fracture of the radius indicated by an arrow.

Case 20

Clinical details

This middle-aged man fell awkwardly onto his outstretched hand. How many fractures are there?

Figure 1. AP wrist.

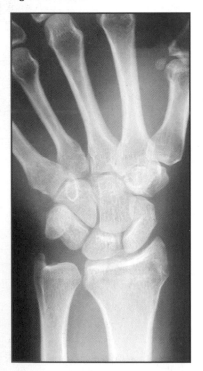

Figure 2. Lateral wrist.

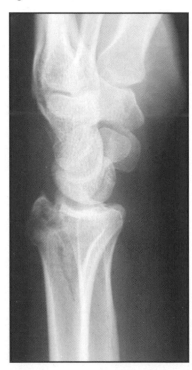

Figure 3. Oblique AP wrist.

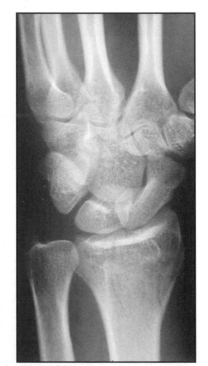

Figure 4. Oblique wrist.

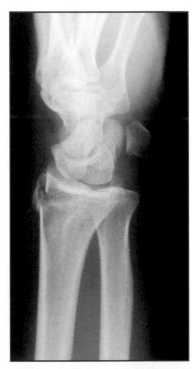

Radiological features

The films presented are scaphoid views, which are designed to highlight fractures of the scaphoid. There are four fractures:

1. a scaphoid fracture
2. a fracture of the distal radius, which involves the articular surface
3. a fracture of the hamate bone (seen on the lateral view, as a small chip of bone lying dorsally)
4. a fracture of the ulnar styloid.

Diagnosis

A fracture of the scaphoid, distal radius, hamate bone and ulnar styloid.

Discussion

The fractures are indicated on the AP and lateral views opposite (Figures 5 and 6, respectively).

Figure 5. The AP view. The scaphoid fracture is indicated by the short arrow and the ulnar fracture is indicated by the long arrow.

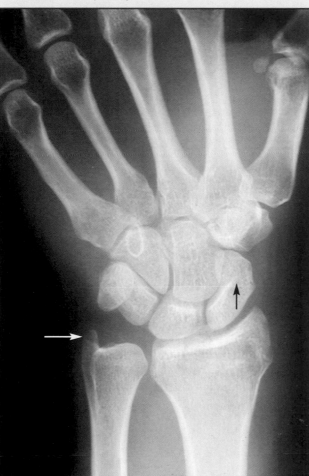

Figure 6. The lateral view with the small chip of bone lying dorsally (hamate fracture) indicated by the small arrow and the radial fracture which involves the joint surface indicated by the long arrow.

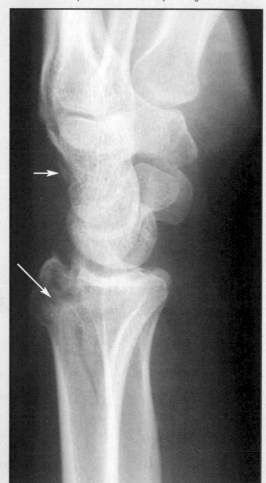

Case 21

Is there anything unusual about this fracture?

Figure 1. AP hand.

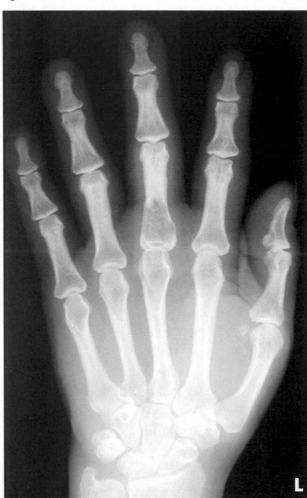

Figure 2. Oblique hand.

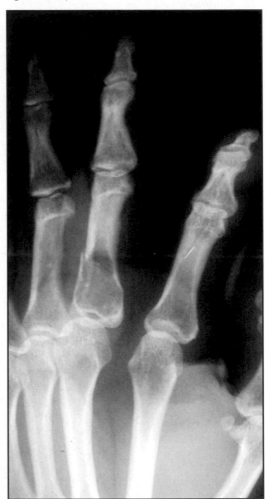

Radiological features

This is a pathological fracture, i.e. through abnormal bone. There is cystic expansion of the proximal phalanx of the middle finger. This could represent several lesions, such as fibrous dysplasia or a simple bone cyst, but its position is typical of an enchondroma, which is benign. The lesion looks benign because it has a narrow zone of transition (the distance between the normal and abnormal regions of the bone) and there is no cortical destruction or periosteal reaction.

Diagnosis

Pathological fracture of proximal phalanx of middle finger.

Discussion

The fracture is indicated on the AP view opposite (Figure 3).

Figure 3. The AP view with the fracture indicated by an arrow.

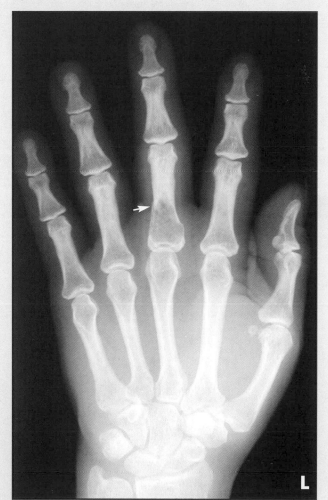

Case 22

Which carpal bone is fractured?

Figure 1. Lateral wrist.

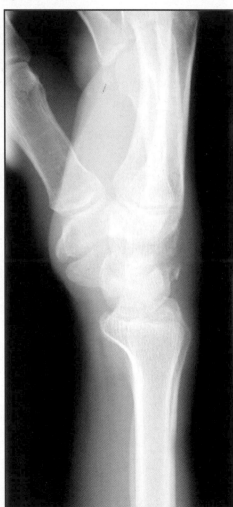

Radiological features

The triquetral is fractured. There is a small fragment of bone lying dorsal to the carpal bones on the lateral view, at a level between the proximal and distal carpal bones. This is most commonly caused by a triquetral fracture.

Diagnosis

Triquetral fracture.

Discussion

Two other examples of triquetral fractures are shown opposite (Figures 2 and 3). Triquetral fractures are the second most common fracture of the wrist after scaphoid fractures.

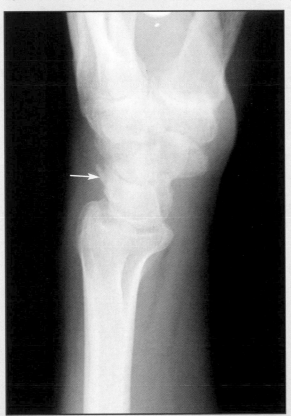

Figure 2. Lateral view with the triquetral fracture indicated by the arrow.

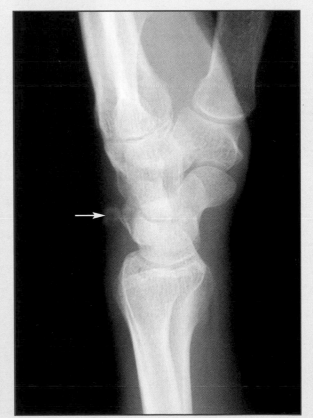

Figure 3. Lateral view with the triquetral fracture indicated by the arrow.

Case 23

Which carpal bone is fractured?

Figure 1. Lateral wrist.

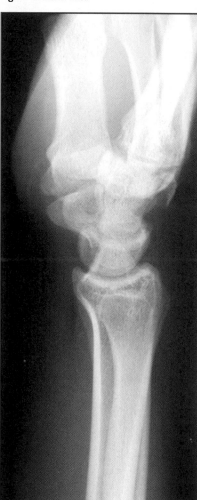

Figure 2. Oblique wrist.

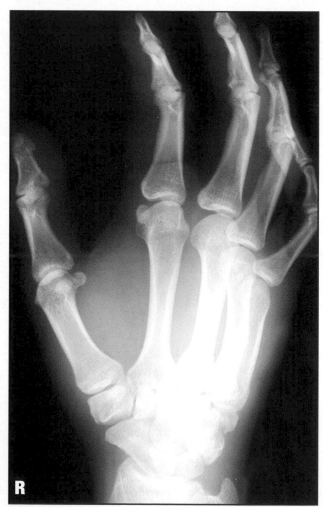

Radiological features

A small fragment of bone is seen lying dorsally to the distal carpal bones. This is due to a fracture of the hamate.

Diagnosis

Fracture of hamate.

Discussion

The fragment of bone is indicated on the lateral view opposite (Figure 3).

Figure 3. The lateral view with the fragment of bone indicated by an arrow.

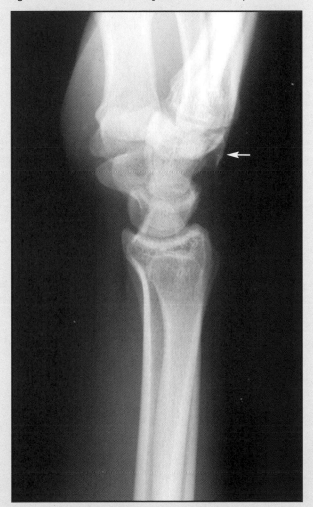

Case Studies

Case 24

Is there a scaphoid fracture?

Figure 1. Lateral wrist.

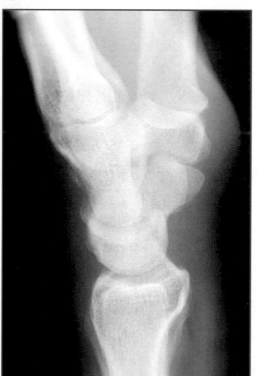

Figure 2. Scaphoid wrist view.

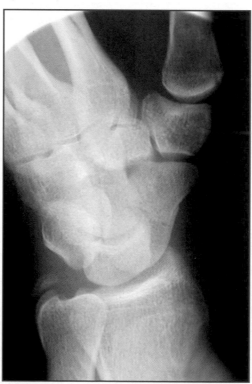

Figure 3. Standard AP wrist.

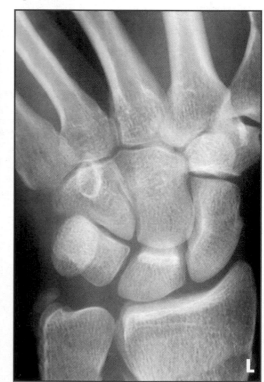

Radiological features

Yes, there is a fracture across the mid-third of the scaphoid, visible on the scaphoid view. Note how it is almost impossible to see the scaphoid fracture on the standard AP and lateral radiographs of the wrist.

Diagnosis

Scaphoid fracture.

Discussion

If a scaphoid fracture is suspected clinically but is not observed on the plain film, then there may be a fracture that is just not yet that apparent. The patient should be placed in a scaphoid cast and re-X-rayed 10 days to 2 weeks later. If no fracture is subsequently observed on plain films but a fracture is still suspected clinically then a bone scan may show a 'hot spot', i.e. a local area of increased uptake of radio-nuclide at a fracture site. Alternatively, an MRI will show bone edema and a fracture line.

The scaphoid fracture in this case, is outlined on the scaphoid view opposite (Figure 4).

Figure 4. The scaphoid view with the fracture outlined.

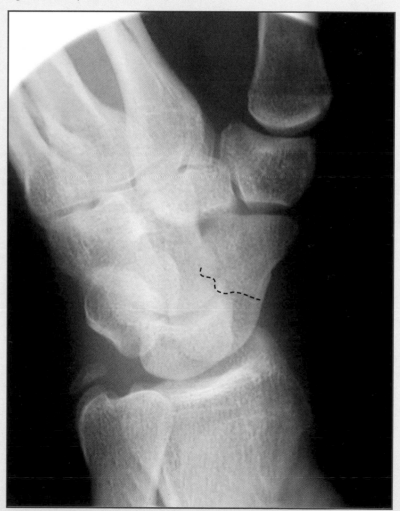

Case 25

Is there a fracture?

Figure 1. AP hand.

Figure 2. Oblique hand.

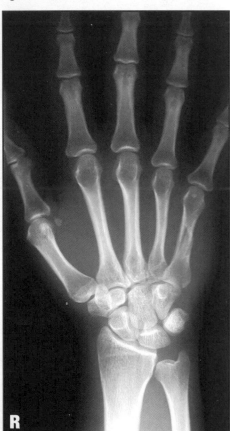

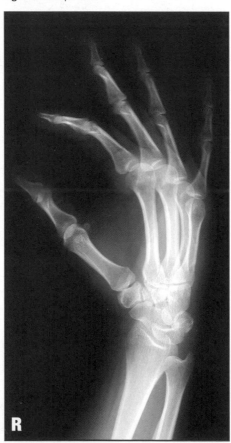

Radiological features

Yes, but it is difficult to see on the oblique view. There is a spiral fracture of the midshaft of the fifth metacarpal, which is well aligned and best seen on the AP view.

Diagnosis

Spiral fracture of the fifth metacarpal.

Case 26

Clinical details
This elderly lady fell in the snow.

Figure 1. Lateral wrist.

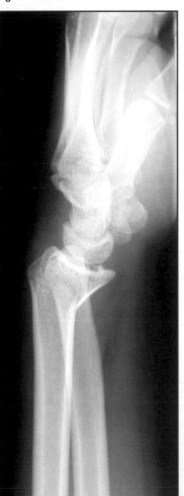

Radiological features
There is a fracture of the distal radius with dorsal angulation and impaction. This is a Colles' fracture. Note the raised pronator fat pad indicating a joint effusion.

Diagnosis
Colles' fracture.

Discussion
The raised fat pad is outlined on the lateral view opposite (Figure 2).

Figure 2. The lateral view with the raised fat pad outlined.

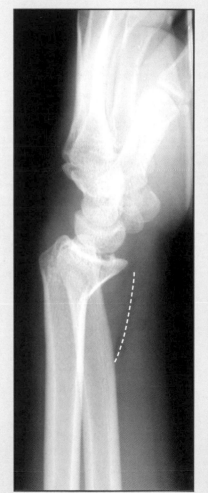

Case Studies

Case 27

Clinical details
This child was refusing to
let anyone touch his hand.

Figure 1. AP hand.

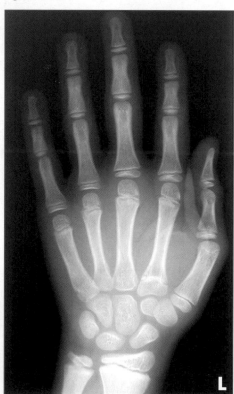

Figure 2. Oblique hand.

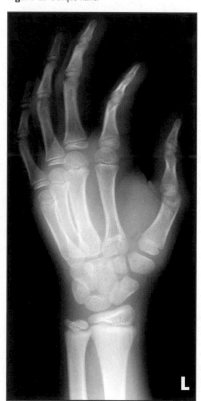

Radiological features
There is a spiral fracture of the
middle finger—this is very hard
to see on the AP view but easier
to see on the oblique.

Diagnosis
Fracture of shaft of the middle
third metacarpal bone.

Case 28

What is the abnormality?

Radiological features

The lunate bone is dislocated in a palmar direction. This is best seen on the lateral view where the capitate, lunate and radius do not line up as they should. However, loss of the normal proximal carpal alignment can also be seen on the AP view.

Diagnosis

Lunate dislocation.

Discussion

The dislocated lunate bone is outlined on the lateral view below (Figure 2).

Figure 1. Lateral and AP wrist.

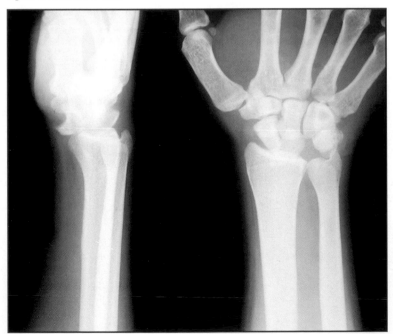

Figure 2. The lateral view with the dislocated lunate bone outlined.

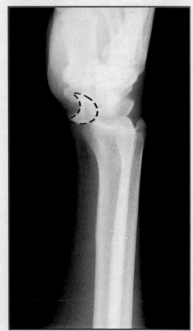

Case 29

Clinical details

This man had tenderness over the anatomical snuff box. What is the injury and what complication can occur?

Figure 1. AP wrist with ulnar deviation.

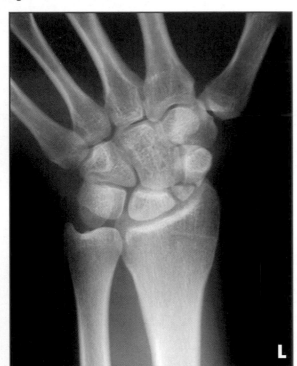

Figure 2. Scaphoid wrist view.

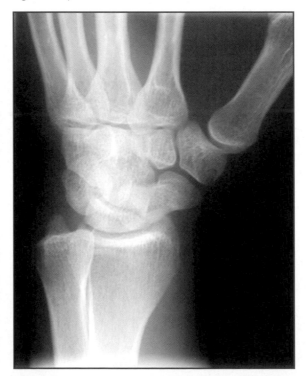

Radiological features

There is a fracture through the proximal third of the scaphoid, which is seen best on the AP view with ulnar deviation.

Diagnosis

Scaphoid fracture.

Discussion

The blood supply of the scaphoid runs distal to proximal. Therefore, a fracture through the waist may result in avascular necrosis (AVN) of the proximal scaphoid. The risk of AVN depends upon the following two properties:

1. displacement of fracture—the risk of AVN increases with greater displacement
2. location of fracture:
   a) fracture of the distal third— fragments usually reunite
   b) fracture of the middle third (the most common site)— failure to reunite occurs in 90%
   c) fracture of the proximal third—failure to reunite occurs in 90%

As this is a fracture through the proximal third of the scaphoid, there is a high chance of non-union.

Case 30

Clinical details
This patient complained of wrist pain after a fall.

Diagnosis
Normal wrist.

Figure 1. AP wrist.

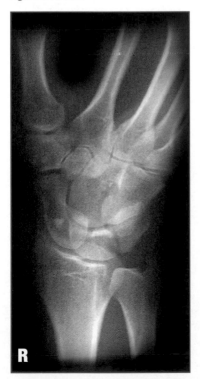

Figure 2. Lateral wrist.

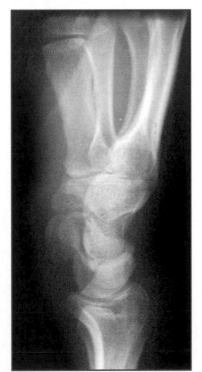

Case 31

Clinical details
This elderly patient fell onto an outstretched hand.

Figure 1. Lateral wrist.

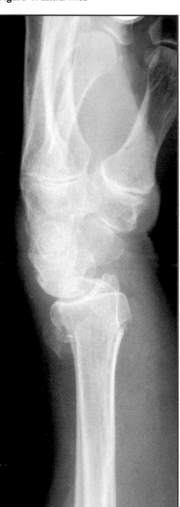

Figure 2. AP wrist.

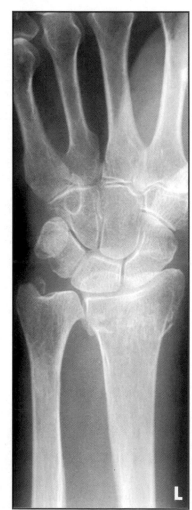

Radiological features
Fracture of the distal radius with dorsal angulation and some impaction of the distal fragment. There is also a fracture of the ulnar styloid, which is a common association. Note the generalized osteopenia.

Diagnosis
Colles' fracture and ulnar styloid fracture.

Case 32

Clinical details
This young man was involved in a fight and was worried that he had broken his hand.

Diagnosis
No fracture.

Figure 1. AP hand.

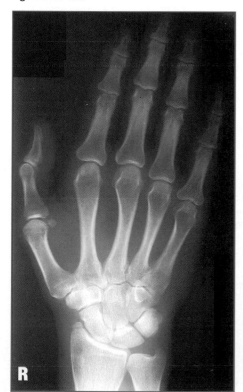

Figure 2. Oblique hand.

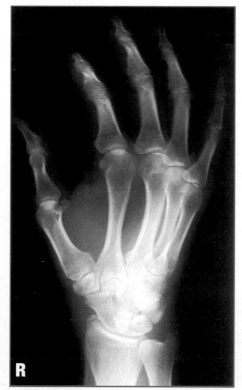

Case Studies

Case 33

Clinical details
This man arrived at the Emergency Department with a painful hand after 'punching a wall'.

Figure 1. AP hand.

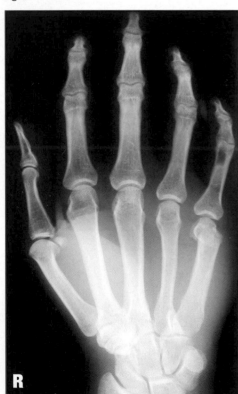

Figure 2. Oblique hand.

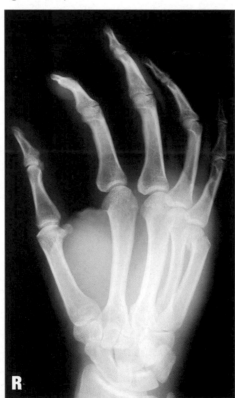

Radiological features
This is a classic boxer's fracture of the distal fifth metacarpal. It does not involve the articular surface, but there is dorsal angulation and the fracture is comminuted.

Diagnosis
Boxer's fracture of the fifth metacarpal.

Discussion
A small degree of angulation can be tolerated in the fourth and fifth metacarpals, because movement of these bones at the carpo-metacarpal joint can compensate for it. This is not true for second and third metacarpal fractures which need to be treated more aggressively.

Case 34

Clinical details
This patient fell and experienced pain over the proximal fifth metacarpal.

Radiological features
This is a tricky one. The alignment between the proximal fourth and fifth metacarpals and the hamate is lost, and these three bones overlap (normally a joint space should be observed between them). This is due to carpo-metacarpal dislocation involving the fourth and fifth metacarpals.

Diagnosis
Carpo-metacarpal dislocation involving fourth and fifth metacarpals.

Discussion
In some cases, this type of injury can be associated with fractures of the base of the metacarpals.

Figure 1. AP hand.

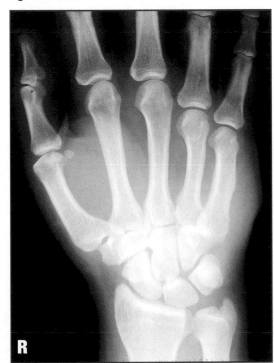

Figure 2. Oblique hand.

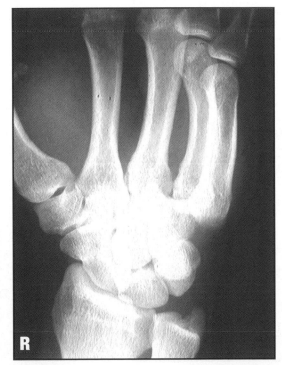

Case 35

What is the mechanism of
injury here?

Figure 1. AP thumb.

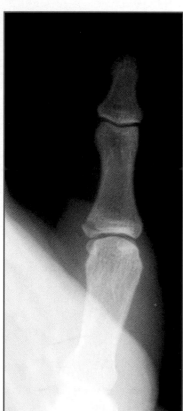

Figure 2. Lateral thumb.

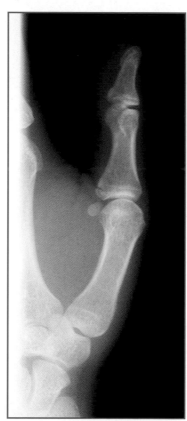

Radiological features

This is a 'gamekeeper's thumb'.
There is rupture of the ulnar
collateral ligament at the first
metacarpophalangeal (MCP) joint.

Diagnosis

Rupture of the ulnar collateral
ligament.

Discussion

In this case, the base of the first
phalanx is avulsed (indicated on the
AP view opposite – see Figure 3).

Rupture of the ulnar collateral
ligament may or may not be
associated with a bony fragment.
If there is no bony fragment, a
radiograph taken in 'abduction
stress' will show that the joint
becomes abnormally wide if the
collateral ligament is torn. A
complete tear is repaired surgically.

Figure 3. The AP view with the avulsion
indicated by an arrow.

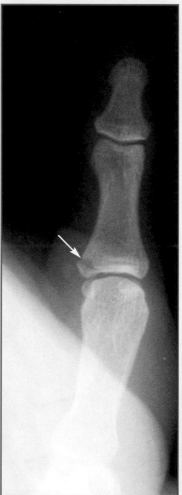

Case 36

What is the abnormality?

Figure 1. AP thumb.

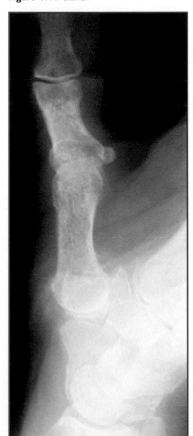

Figure 2. Lateral thumb.

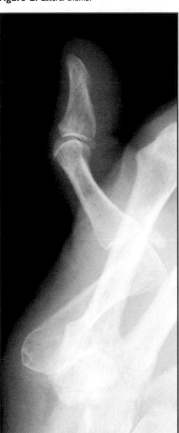

Radiological features

These films underline how important it is to have two views at right angles to each other—only on the lateral view of the thumb does it become apparent how malaligned the metacarpal and phalanx are.

Diagnosis

Dislocation at the first MCP joint and malalignment at the first carpo-metacarpal joint.

Case 37

Case 37

What is this fracture? How should it be managed?

Figure 1. AP hand.

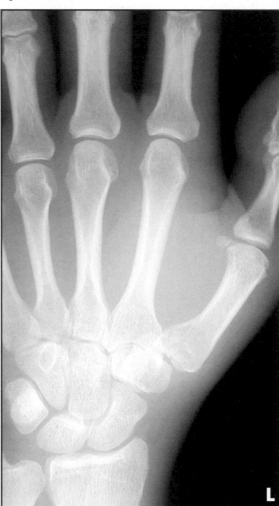

Figure 2. Oblique hand.

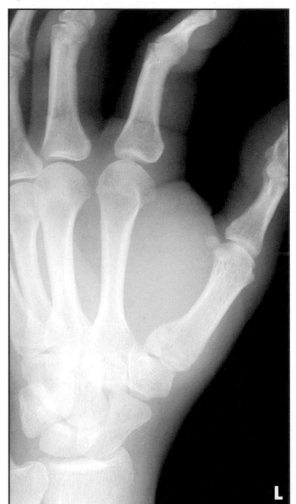

Radiological features

There is a fracture of the base of the first metacarpal extending to the joint surface.

Diagnosis

Bennett's fracture (of the base of the first metacarpal).

Discussion

Although there is little displacement in this example, dislocation of the fragment can often occur because the unopposed action of the abductor pollicis longus muscle pulls the metacarpal (but not the free fragment) laterally. It is important to reduce this fracture to the anatomical position. Open reduction and internal fixation is often necessary as it is difficult to maintain anatomical alignment.

The fracture is outlined on the AP view opposite (Figure 3).

Figure 3. The AP view with the fracture outlined.

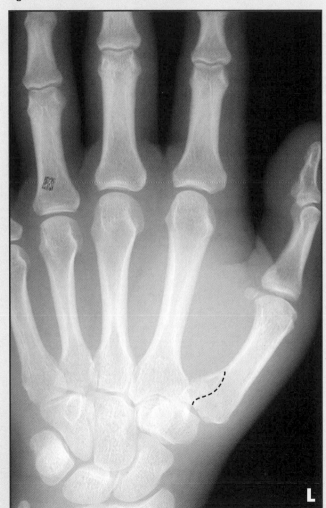

Case 38

What is the abnormality?

Figure 1. AP hand.

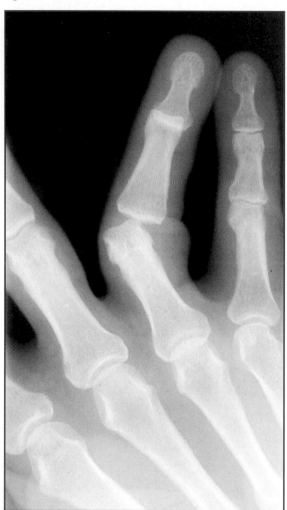

Figure 2. Lateral hand.

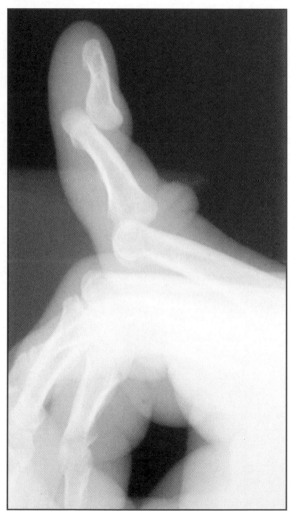

Diagnosis

Dislocation at the proximal interphalangeal and distal interphalangeal joints of the ring finger.

Discussion

The reduced AP and lateral views are shown opposite (Figures 3 and 4, respectively).

Figure 3. The reduced AP view.

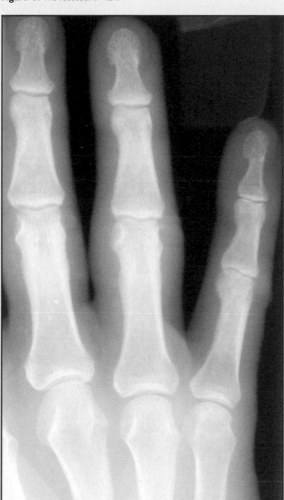

Figure 4. The reduced lateral view.

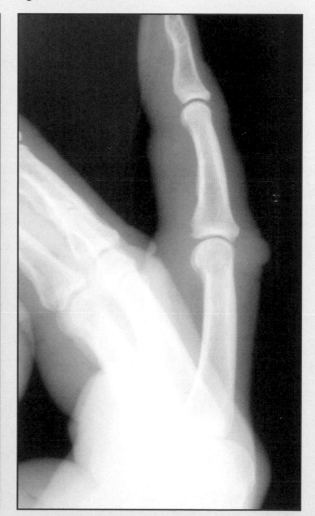

Lower Limb

Rules and Tools

Introduction

The lower limb incorporates the following areas: the hip, knee, ankle and foot. Radiographic projections are mainly anteroposterior (AP), horizontal beam lateral (HBL) and lateral, plus dorsoplantar (DP) and oblique for the foot.

Hip

Hip views
- AP (most useful)
- Lateral

Film-viewing routine
AP view (Figures 1 and 2)
Check:
- Shenton's line (see line 1, Figure 1) —follow Shenton's line along the medial aspect of the femoral shaft and neck, to the inferior aspect of the superior pubic ramus (if in doubt compare to the opposite side); any discontinuity suggests a fracture of the femoral neck
- the trabecular pattern of the neck of the femur—it should be continuous (Figure 2); if not, suspect a fracture
- the inferior and superior pubic rami for fractures—injuries in these areas are a common cause of hip pain when a fracture of the neck of the femur has been ruled out

Lateral view
Check:
- a line drawn through the middle of the femoral neck passes through the femoral head; if not suspect a fracture

Figure 1. AP view of the hip.

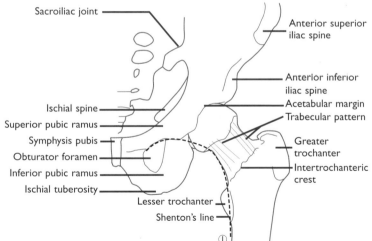

Sacroiliac joint

Anterior superior
iliac spine

Anterior inferior
iliac spine

Ischial spine
Superior pubic ramus
Symphysis pubis
Obturator foramen
Inferior pubic ramus
Ischial tuberosity

Acetabular margin
Trabecular pattern

Greater
trochanter

Intertrochanteric
crest

Lesser trochanter
Shenton's line

Figure 2. AP radiograph to show normal trabecular pattern.

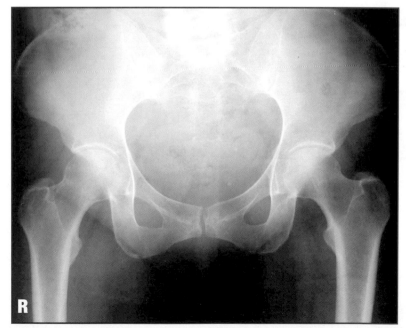

Knee

Knee views
- HBL
- AP

Film-viewing routine

HBL view (Figures 3a and 3b)
Look for:
- a fat–fluid level (lipohemarthrosis) —this is visible as a black region (fat) above a whiter fluid level (blood). It is caused by an intraarticular fracture, leading to release of blood and bone marrow fat into the joint space (as can be seen in Figures 3a and 3b)
- soft-tissue swelling in the supra-patellar region, due to an effusion

AP view (Figures 4a and 4b)
Look for:
- soft-tissue swelling, due to an effusion
- depressions in the surface of the tibial plateau

Look at:
- the cortical outline of the femur, tibia and fibula to identify any breaks

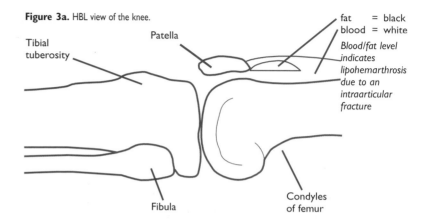

Figure 3a. HBL view of the knee.

Tibial tuberosity

Patella

fat = black
blood = white

Blood/fat level indicates lipohemarthrosis due to an intraarticular fracture

Fibula

Condyles of femur

Figure 3b. Fat-fluid level/lipohemarthrosis.

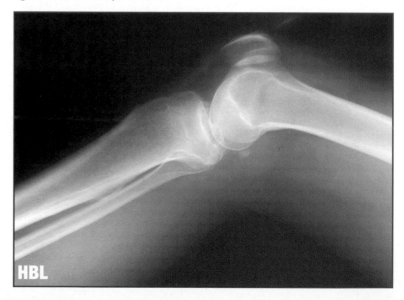

HBL

Additional information

If there is a fracture of the lower tibia or fibula, an X-ray of the knee must be taken as well. The tibia and fibula act as a ring. Therefore, if a fracture is seen involving one site within the ring, consider a fracture occurring elsewhere within the ring.

Figure 4a. AP view of the knee.

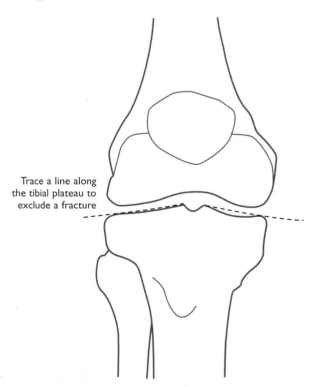

Trace a line along the tibial plateau to exclude a fracture

Figure 4b. Normal AP radiograph of the knee.

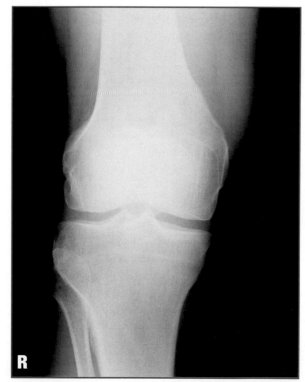

Ankle

Ankle views
- AP
- Lateral

Film-viewing routine
AP view (Figures 5a and 5b)
Look for:
- soft-tissue swelling in the medial and lateral soft-tissues—this commonly occurs without a fracture and is due to ligamentous injury

Check:
- along the cortical edge of the fibula and tibia for fractures
- the space between the fibula, tibia and talus is symmetrical; otherwise suspect a talar dome fracture

Lateral view (Figures 6a and 6b)
Look for:
- continuity of the trabecular pattern within the calcaneum; suspect a fracture if any irregularities are present

Look at:
- the base of the fifth metatarsal—presence of a fracture here can be a cause of lateral ankle pain
- Bohler's angle (illustrated in Figure 7 and in Case 14); if it is not between 20–40°, suspect a calcaneal fracture

Figure 5a. AP view of the ankle.

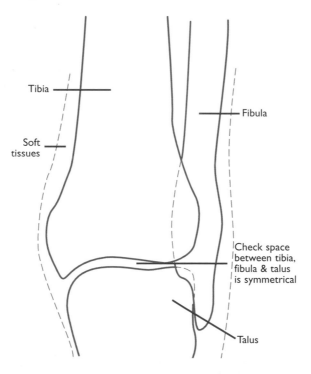

Tibia

Fibula

Soft tissues

Check space between tibia, fibula & talus is symmetrical

Talus

Figure 5b. Normal AP radiograph of the ankle.

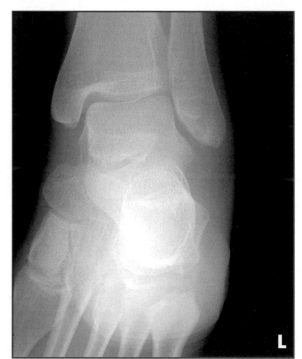

L

Additional information

- There are many accessory ossicles in the foot and ankle. An ossicle is usually well-defined (i.e. it has a sclerotic/corticated outline) but a fracture fragment usually does not have a cortex around all of its margins
- A calcaneal fracture may be associated with fractures of the spine or pelvis since the force causing the calcaneal fracture is transmitted upwards; therefore an X-ray of the spine and pelvis may need to be taken as well

Figure 6a. Lateral view of the ankle.

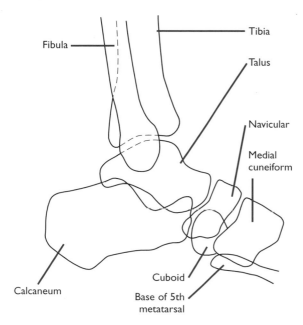

Fibula

Tibia

Talus

Navicular

Medial cuneiform

Calcaneum

Cuboid

Base of 5th metatarsal

Figure 6b. Normal lateral radiograph of the ankle.

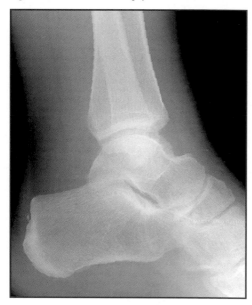

Figure 7. Bohler's angle.

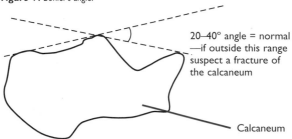

20–40° angle = normal —if outside this range suspect a fracture of the calcaneum

Calcaneum

Foot

Foot view

- DP
- Oblique

Film-viewing routine

*Dorsal (Figures 8a and 8b)
and oblique views*

Look:

- along the cortical edge of the bones to exclude a break
- for tarso–metatarsal dislocation (Lisfranc fracture dislocation)— the lateral edge of the first metatarsal should align with the lateral edge of the medial cuneiform, the medial border of the second metatarsal should align with the medial border of the intermediate/middle cuneiform and the lateral edge of the fourth metatarsal should align with the lateral border of the cuboid (see also Discussion to Case 16); if these alignments are lost, suspect a tarso–metatarsal dislocation

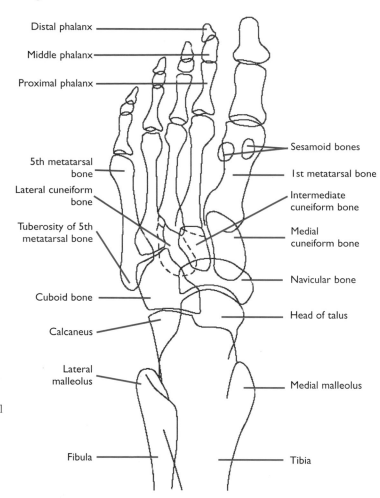

Figure 8a. DP view of the foot.

Distal phalanx

Middle phalanx

Proximal phalanx

5th metatarsal bone

Lateral cuneiform bone

Tuberosity of 5th metatarsal bone

Cuboid bone

Calcaneus

Lateral malleolus

Fibula

Sesamoid bones

1st metatarsal bone

Intermediate cuneiform bone

Medial cuneiform bone

Navicular bone

Head of talus

Medial malleolus

Tibia

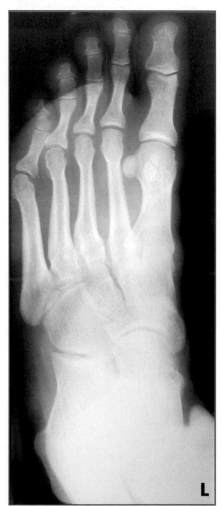

Figure 8b. Normal DP radiograph of the foot.

L

Case Studies

Case 1

Clinical details
This elderly patient slipped on ice and was unable to stand again due to hip pain.

Figure 1. AP hip.

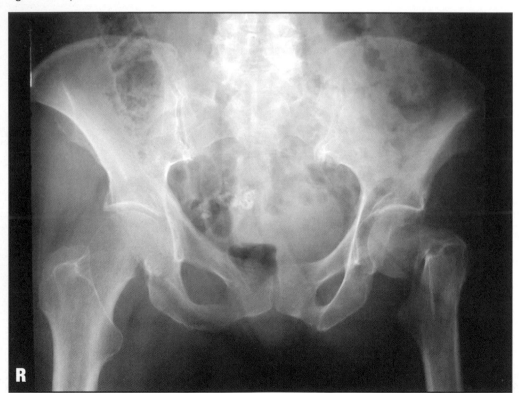

Figure 2. Lateral hip.

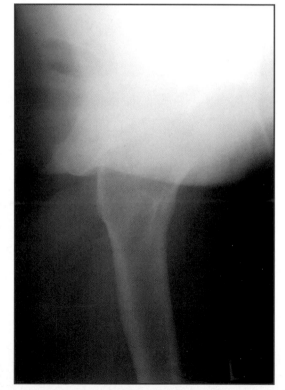

Radiological features

There is a sub-capital fracture of the left femoral neck which is more easily visible on the AP than the lateral view. There is loss of the continuity of Shenton's line on the left side.

Diagnosis

Left sub-capital femoral neck fracture.

Discussion

Shenton's line is intact on the right side, but not on the left (Figure 3).

Figure 3. The AP view. The normal Shenton's line is outlined on the right side.

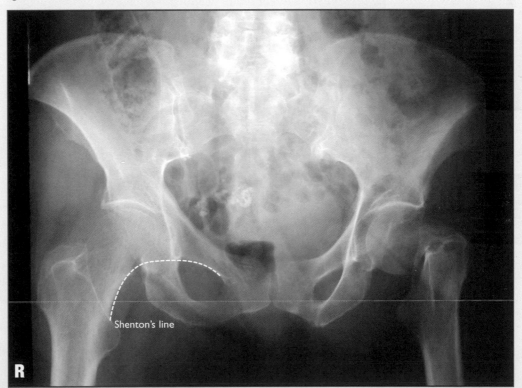

Shenton's line

R

Case 2

Clinical details

This patient complained of multifocal bone pain for several months and an acute onset of pain in the right hip after an innocuous injury.

Figure 1. AP hip.

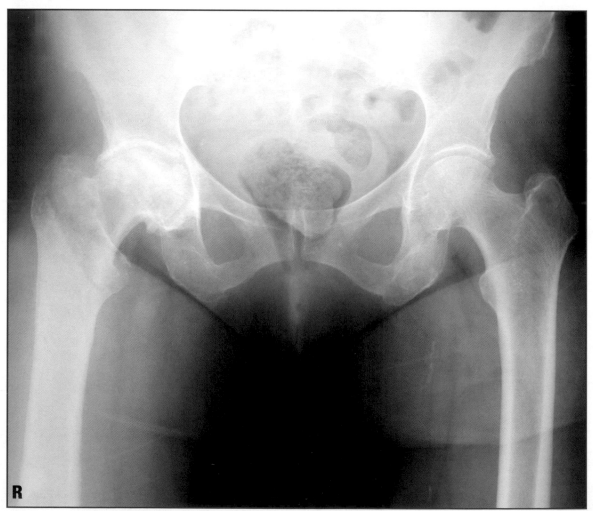

Radiological features

There is a per trochanteric fracture of the right femur, with slight distraction of the fracture's fragments.

In addition to the fracture, there is abnormal texture of the shaft of the right femur with medullary cavity expansion, cortical thickening and sclerosis—all features of Paget's disease of the bone.

Severe unilateral degenerate changes are present in the right hip joint: loss of joint space; articular sclerosis; subarticular cyst formation (focal rounded lucencies immediately below the articular surface); and osteophyte formation.

Diagnosis

Right per trochanteric femoral fracture.

Discussion

Although there is sclerosis and cortical thickening in Paget's disease, the bone texture overall is abnormal and more likely to fracture than normal bone. The trochanteric fracture is outlined on the AP view (Figure 2).

Figure 2. The AP view with the fracture outlined. (Note also the difference in bone texture of both femurs.)

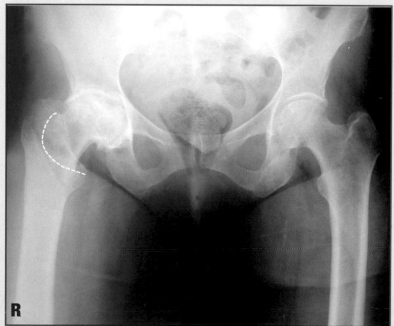

Case Studies

Case 3

Clinical details
This elderly lady had pain in her hip after falling on an uneven pavement. The limb did not appear significantly shortened.

Radiological features
There is discontinuity of Shenton's line on the left with an impaction fracture of the left neck of the femur.

Diagnosis
Fracture of left neck of femur.

Figure 1. AP hip.

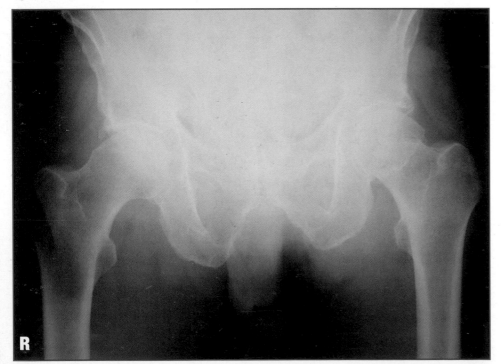

Case 4

Clinical details
This 65-year-old lady fell over
and complained of bruising and
pain in her knee.

Radiological features
There is no soft-tissue swelling
and no fracture. The intercondylar
tibial spines are spiked due to
degenerative disease.

Diagnosis
No fracture.

Figure 1. AP knee.

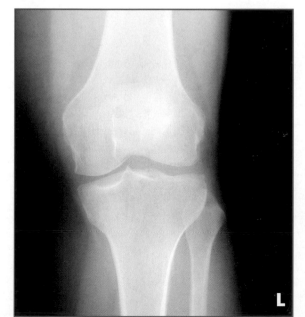

Figure 2. Lateral knee.

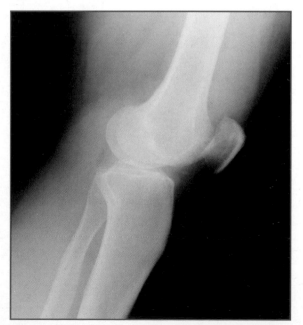

Case 5

Clinical details

This patient fell off a mountain bike. Shortly after arriving in hospital, the patient became increasingly short of breath and was clinically shocked. A central line was inserted and a chest X-ray (CXR) was taken to exclude a pneumothorax or chest wall injury as the cause. How would you describe the abnormalities and what are the possible causes?

Figure 1. Lateral view of femoral shaft.

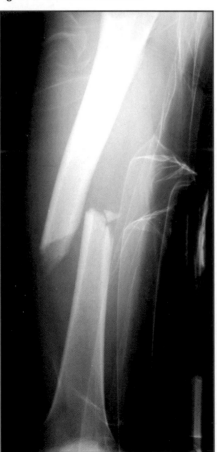

Figure 2. Frontal CXR.

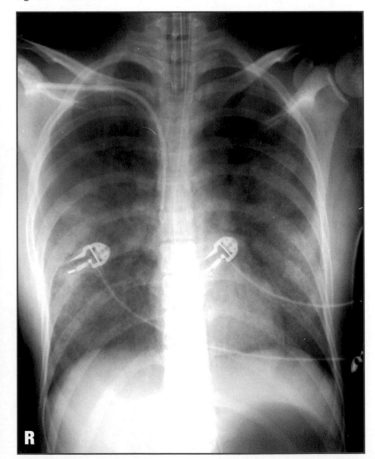

Radiological features

There is a displaced spiral fracture
of the mid-femur.

On the CXR, there is
ill-defined nodular shadowing
throughout both lungs,
predominating in the mid-zones
and bases. No chest wall injury
or pneumothorax is present.

Diagnosis

Spiral fracture of the mid-femur
complicated by fat embolism.

Discussion

The medulla of the long bones in
adulthood contains fatty marrow.
Therefore, as a result of the
fracture, the fat may enter the
venous circulation and, after passing
through the right-sided cardiac
chambers, become lodged in the
pulmonary circulation. This has
a high mortality rate.

Case Studies

Case 6

Clinical details

This woman was pushed to the
ground and on trying to stand she
felt something 'give' in her knee.
She was unable to straighten her
leg voluntarily.

Figure 1. AP knee.

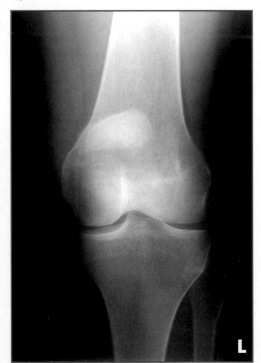

Figure 2. Lateral knee.

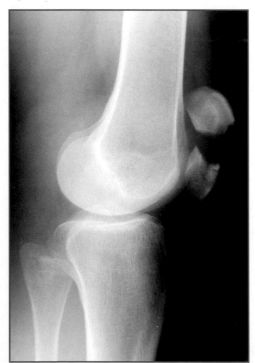

Radiological features

There is a horizontal fracture of
the lower part of the patella.

Diagnosis

Patellar fracture.

Discussion

The fracture of the lower part of
the patella interrupts the
quadriceps/patella complex and so
extension of the knee is impossible.
This injury generally requires
surgical intervention.

Case 7

Clinical details
This pedestrian was struck by a speeding car. He complained of pain and swelling in his upper calf, where the car bumper hit him.

Radiological features
There are displaced overlapping fractures of the upper left tibia and fibula.

Diagnosis
Fracture of the proximal left tibia and fibula.

Discussion
The tibia is susceptible to the following mechanisms of injury:
1. torsional stress
2. severe force from, for example, a fall from height or a road traffic accident (RTA)
3. a direct blow from, for example, an RTA or an injury from a falling heavy object.

Figure 1. AP knee.

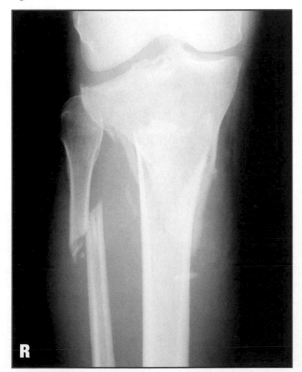

Figure 2. Lateral knee.

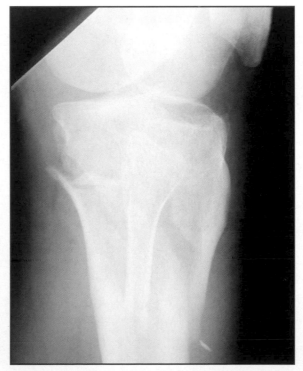

Case 8

Clinical details

This female gymnast landed
awkwardly and immediately felt
severe pain in her left knee.

Figure 1. AP knee.

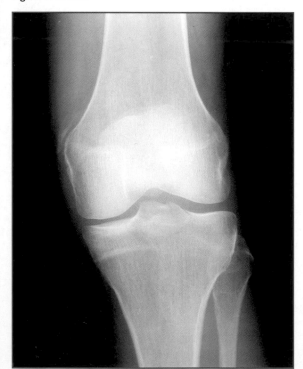

Figure 2. HBL knee.

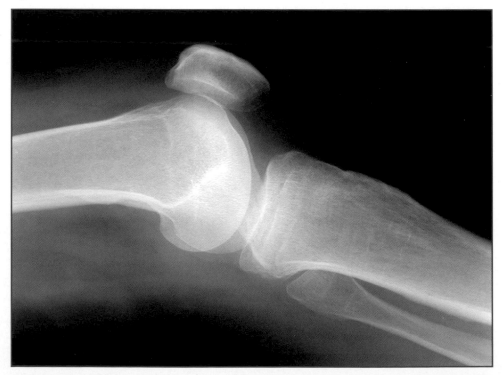

Radiological features

There is a fracture at the base of the left tibial spines. This extends to the posterior surface of the tibia on the horizontal beam lateral (HBL) view. There is increased soft-tissue density in the supra-patellar region, which is visible on the HBL view.

Diagnosis

Fracture of the left tibial spines with a supra-patellar effusion.

Discussion

The increased soft-tissue density in the supra-patellar region is due to a large effusion in the knee joint. The tibial spines are extraarticular and the effusion in this case is 'sympathetic'. If intraarticular structures are fractured, a lipohemarthrosis may result.

The fracture is outlined on both the AP and HBL views opposite (Figures 3 and 4, respectively).

Figure 3. The AP view with fracture and the supra-patellar effusion outlined.

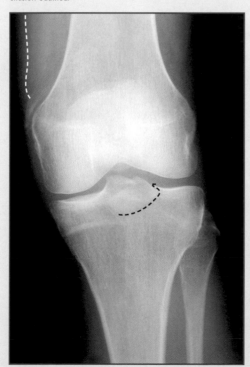

Figure 4. The HBL view with the fracture and the supra-patellar effusion outlined.

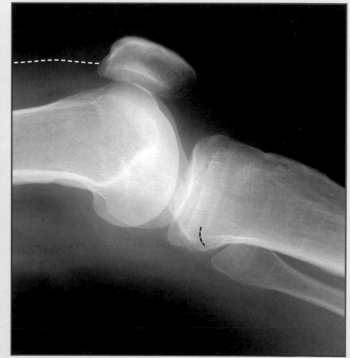

Case 9

Clinical details

This athletic adolescent was experiencing long-standing, intermittent, low intensity pain in his knee for several months.

Figure 1. AP knee.

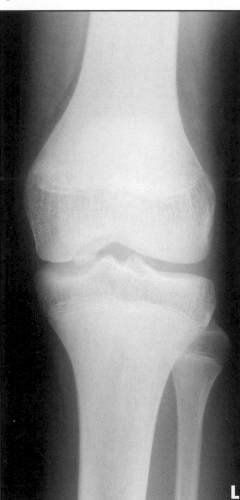

Figure 2. Lateral knee.

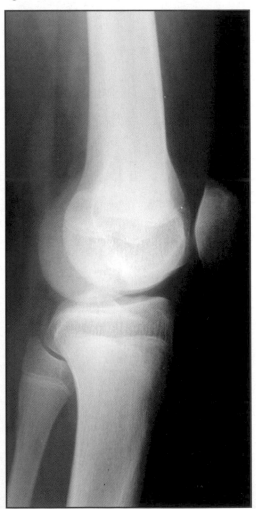

Radiological features

There is an elliptical fragment of bone at the lateral aspect of the medial femoral condyle. This is an osteochondritis dissecans lesion.

Diagnosis

Osteochondritis dissecans defect of the lateral aspect of the medial femoral condyle.

Discussion

An osteochondritis dissecans lesion is thought to be a result of repetitive impaction, which leads to avascular necrosis; the subsequent avascular bone separates from the underlying viable bone. The 'fragment' may remain appropriately sited and still covered with cartilage and synovium, or may migrate and become an intraarticular 'loose body'.

The lesion is outlined on both the AP and lateral views opposite (Figures 3 and 4, respectively).

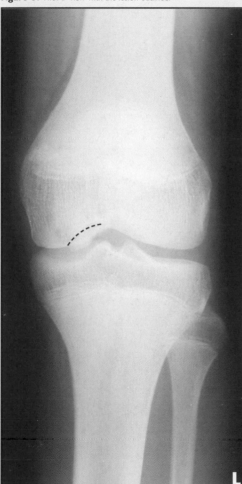

Figure 3. The AP view with the lesion outlined.

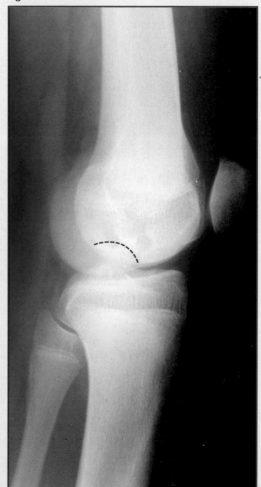

Figure 4. The lateral view with the lesion outlined.

Case 10

Clinical details

This patient was struck on the lateral aspect of his left knee by the bumper of a vehicle. This resulted in severe valgus stress. What radiographic features are present?

Figure 1. AP knee.

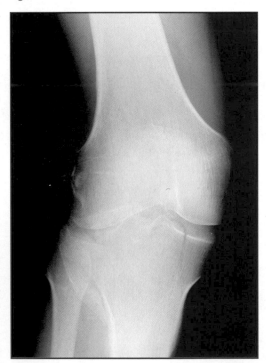

Figure 2. HBL knee.

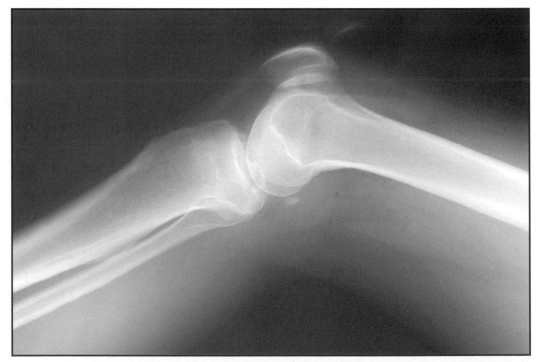

Radiological features

There are fractures of the left tibial spines, left lateral tibial plateau and left medial tibia. On the lateral film, (taken with a horizontal beam parallel to the table-top), there is a fat-fluid level (lipohemarthrosis) in the left supra-patellar bursa and a small fracture fragment seen in the dependant position of the joint posteriorly.

Diagnosis

Left intraarticular fracture with lipohemarthrosis.

Discussion

The fat-fluid level is the result of bone marrow fat separating above the joint effusion/hemorrhage. The presence of a fat-fluid level implies an intraarticular fracture.

The fat-fluid level and the fractures are outlined on the HBL and AP views (Figures 3 and 4, respectively).

Figure 4. The AP view with the fracture of the left tibial spines, left lateral tibial plateau and left medial tibia outlined.

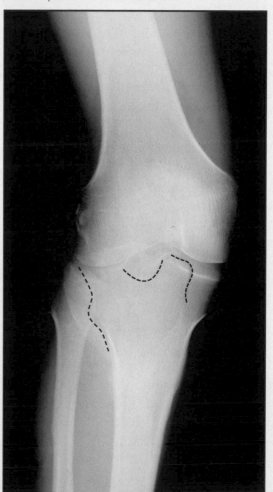

Figure 3. The HBL view with the fat-fluid level outlined.

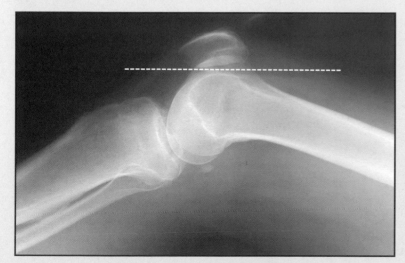

Case 11

Clinical details

This young rugby player was tackled with a sudden onset of pain around his right knee. However, despite the uncomfortable pain, he finished the last 15 minutes of the game. The pain grew worse overnight.

Figure 1. AP knee.

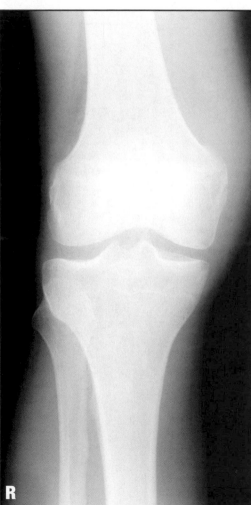

Figure 2. Lateral knee.

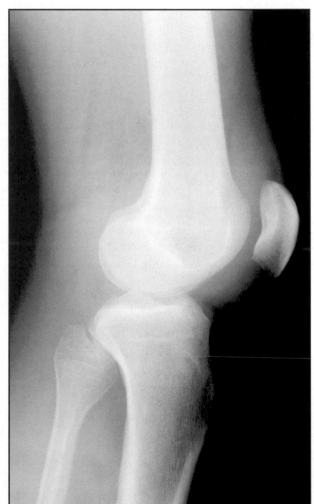

Radiological features

There is an increase in the size and density of the soft-tissue around the right knee joint, due to a large joint effusion. However, no fracture is evident. This effusion is best seen on the lateral view, where rounded soft-tissue density widens the patella-femoral distance. This effusion is also seen on the AP view as increased soft-tissue density, superomedial to the medial femoral condyle.

Diagnosis

Right large knee joint effusion.

Discussion

The effusion is outlined on the lateral view opposite (Figure 3).

Figure 3. The lateral view with the effusion outlined.

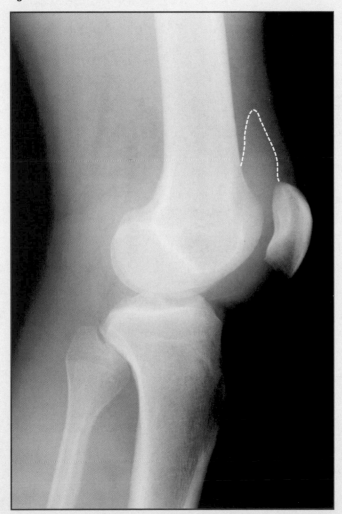

Case 12

Clinical details

This young man stumbled down the stairs after an excessive Friday night's drinking. He felt his ankle twist and was unable to weight-bear.

Figure 1. AP ankle.

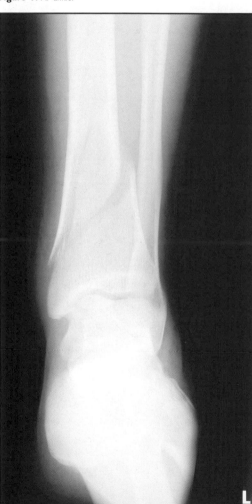

Figure 2. Lateral ankle.

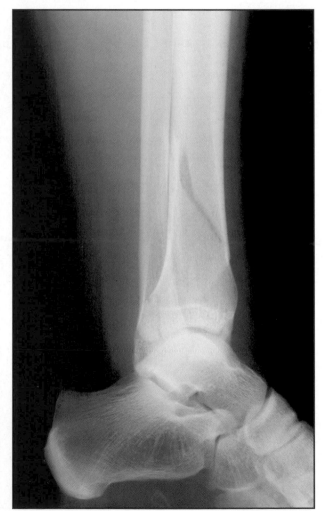

Radiological features

There is a spiral fracture of the distal tibia and an avulsion fracture of the posterior malleolus (posterior tibia).

Diagnosis

Bi-malleolar fracture.

Discussion

The fractures are outlined on the lateral view opposite (Figure 3).

Figure 3. The lateral view with the fractures outlined.

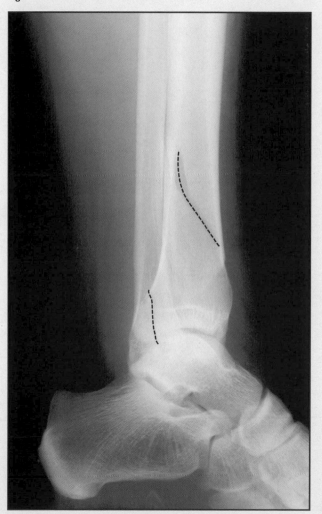

Case 13

Clinical details
This patient landed awkwardly whilst playing basketball. He could not weight-bear and complained of severe pain in his ankle. What do these radiographs show and what further imaging would be sensible?

Figure 1. AP ankle.

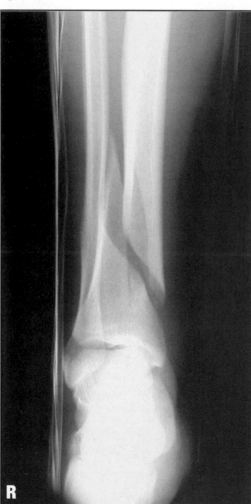

Figure 2. Lateral ankle.

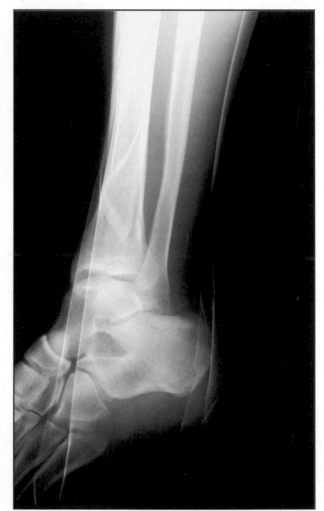

Radiological features

There is a spiral fracture of the distal tibia.

Diagnosis

Fracture of the distal tibia.

Discussion

The spiral fracture of the distal tibia implies a rotational torsional force.

The tibia and fibula in principle act in concert as a ring structure and therefore a second fracture should be looked for. A radiograph including the whole tibia and fibula is necessary. In this case, the knee radiograph demonstrates the spiral fracture of the upper fibula (Figure 3).

Figure 3. HBL knee.

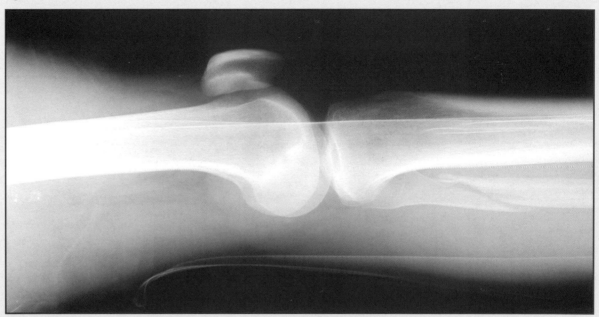

Case 14

Clinical details

This window cleaner fell from his ladder and sustained an injury to his ankle.

Figure 1. Lateral ankle.

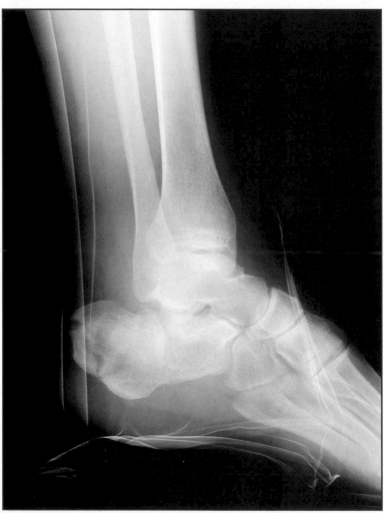

Radiological features

There is a fracture of the body of the right calcaneum, which does not involve the subtalar joint. Bohler's angle is reduced.

Diagnosis

Fractured right calcaneum.

Discussion

This fracture is also seen on the sagittal CT scan (Figure 2).

Bohler's angle lies between a line drawn from the anterior articular process of the calcaneum through the posterior articular surface and the intersecting second line that touches the superior angle of the calcaneal tuberosity and the posterior articular process of the calcaneum (Figure 3). Normally, this angle is between 20–40°. It is decreased in fractures that flatten the heel profile.

Figure 2. Sagittal CT scan through calcaneum.

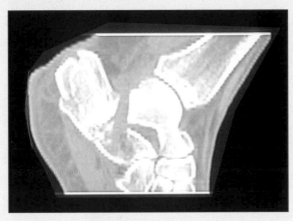

Figure 3. Bohler's angle.

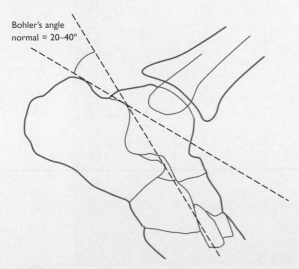

Bohler's angle normal = 20–40°

Case Studies

Case 15

Clinical details

This builder fell 6 m from
scaffolding. He complained of pain
in his right ankle.

Figure 1. Lateral ankle.

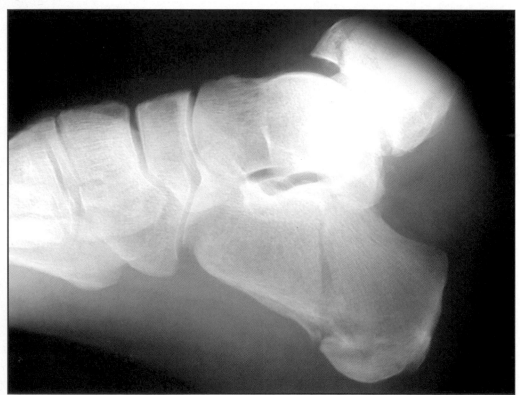

Radiological features

There is a fracture of the body of the right calcaneum extending to involve the subtalar joint and a fracture of the anterior articular surface of the right tibia.

Diagnosis

Right calcaneal fracture and right tibial fracture.

Discussion

The calcaneal fracture was caused by an axial loading injury on the calcaneum, and the forced dorsiflexion of the ankle joint caused the anterior articular fracture of the tibia. The fractures are outlined on the lateral view opposite (Figure 2).

This force also causes injuries of the lower limb, pelvis, spine (dorsolumbar fractures are present in 5% of calcaneal fractures) and the contralateral ankle/calcaneum. Therefore, full clinical (and if necessary radiological) assessment of these areas is mandatory.

Figure 2. The lateral view with the fractures outlined.

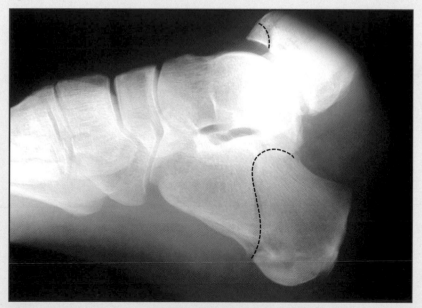

Case 16

Clinical details
This diabetic patient tripped, forcing her forefoot into plantar flexion. Describe the abnormalities.

(Radiographs courtesy of Dr C Prendegast)

Radiological features
There is a fracture of the proximal shaft of the third metatarsal and lateral shift of the second to the fifth metatarsal bases, which overlie the adjacent tarsal bones, implying ligamentous injury. This is described as a Lisfranc fracture dislocation.

Diagnosis
Lisfranc fracture dislocation.

Discussion
The normal tarso-metatarsal joint alignment, outlined below, must be understood clearly to evaluate these ligamentous and bony injuries:

1. the lateral aspect of the first metatarsal aligns with the lateral aspect of the medial cuneiform (on the DP view)
2. the lateral aspect of the second metatarsal aligns with the lateral aspect of the middle cuneiform (on the oblique view)
3. the lateral aspect of the third metatarsal aligns with the lateral aspect of the lateral cuneiform (on the oblique view)
4. the fourth and fifth metatarsals align with the articular surface of the cuboid (on both DP and oblique views).

Figure 1. DP foot.

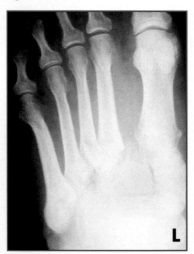

Figure 2. DP oblique foot.

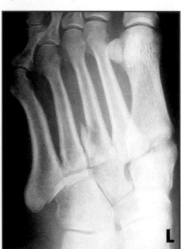

Case 17

Clinical details

A workman dropped a desk on to his toes with extensive bruising, but he was able to weight-bear.

Radiological features

There is disruption of the trabecular pattern of the proximal half of the distal phalanx of the left great toe.

Diagnosis

Crush fracture of the left great toe.

Figure 1. Lateral great toe.

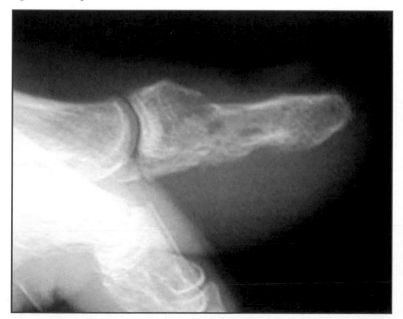

Figure 2. DP great toe.

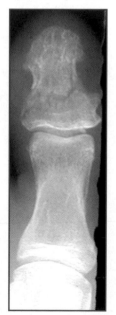

Case 18

Clinical details
This patient tripped while dancing.

Figure 1. DP toes.

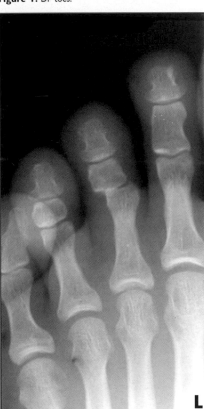

Figure 2. DP oblique toes.

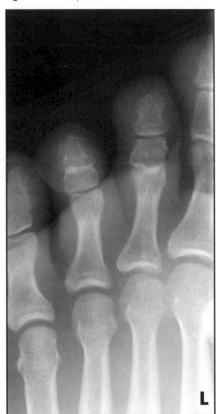

Radiological features
There is incongruity of the articular surfaces of the bones of the proximal interphalangeal joint of the left third toe, which implies ligamentous injury and lateral subluxation.

Diagnosis
Interphalangeal joint dislocation of the left third toe.

Case 19

Clinical details
This patient stubbed his toes and
had extensive bruising.

Figure 1. AP foot.

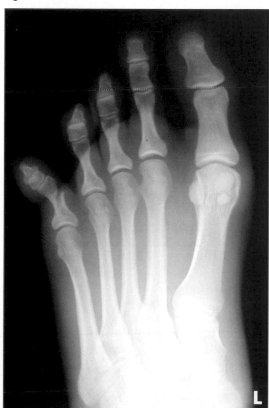

Figure 2. Oblique foot.

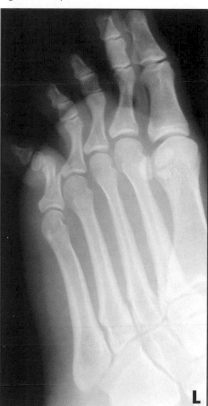

Radiological features
There is an angulated oblique
fracture of the proximal phalanx
of the left little toe, with adjacent
soft-tissue swelling.

Diagnosis
Fracture of the left fifth proximal
phalanx.

Case 20

Case 20

Clinical details
This young man had a swollen,
painful ankle after falling off a wall.

Figure 1. AP ankle.

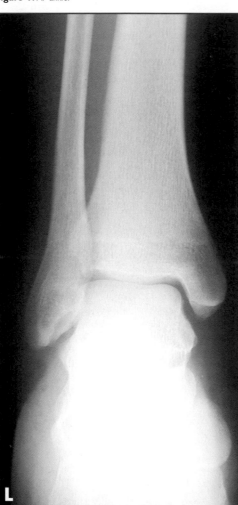

Figure 2. Lateral ankle.

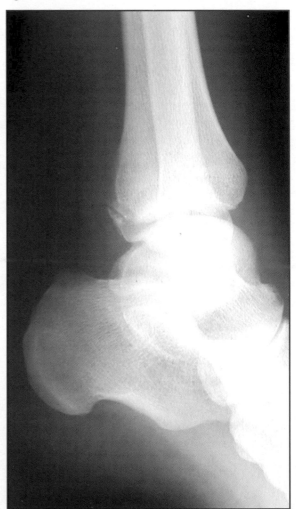

Radiological features

There is soft-tissue swelling and a fracture of the posterior tibia.

Diagnosis

Posterior tibial fracture.

Discussion

The posterior tibia is the 'third' malleolus and it is quite rare to see a fracture of the posterior tibia without fractures to the medial and lateral malleoli as well.

Fractures of the ankle are classified according to the following mechanisms (Figure 3):

1. **adduction/inversion** causes a transverse fracture of the lateral malleolus and an oblique fracture of the medial malleolus
2. **inversion and external rotation** causes an oblique fracture of the fibula and a posterior tibial fracture
3. **eversion** causes a transverse fracture of the medial malleolus and an oblique fracture of the lateral malleolus, plus a posterior tibial fracture if externally rotated
4. **forced dorsiflexion** causes a comminuted fracture of the tibial plafond and distal fibula.

Figure 3. Illustrations of fractures of the ankle.

a) Adduction/inversion

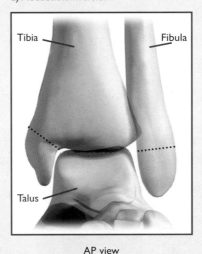

AP view

b) Inversion and external rotation

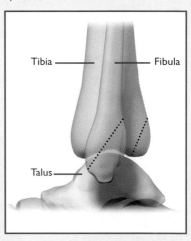

Lateral view

c) Eversion

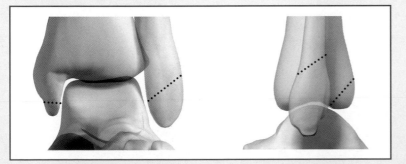

AP view   Lateral view

d) Forced dorsiflexion

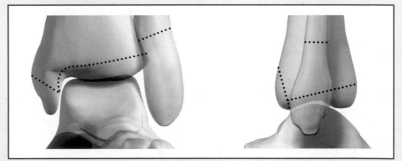

AP view   Lateral view

Case Studies

Case 21

Clinical details
This patient fell from a motorbike. What are the radiological features and what is the likely mechanism of injury?

Figure 1. AP ankle.

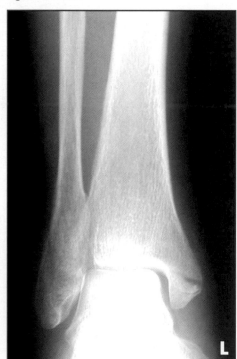

Figure 2. Lateral ankle.

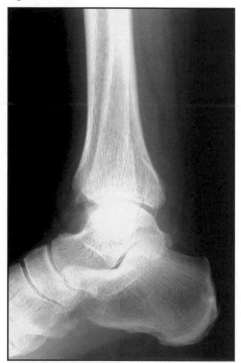

Radiological features
There is a distal third fracture of the right fibula, and a fracture of the medial malleolus. The lateral joint space between the lateral malleolus and lateral aspect of the talus is widened.

Diagnosis
Right distal fibula shaft and medial malleolus fracture.

Discussion
These injuries are caused by forced inversion and plantar flexion. The widening of joint space between the lateral malleolus and lateral aspect of the talus may imply disruption of the lateral ligament complex that attaches the distal fibula to both the talus and calcaneum.

In cases of complex ankle trauma, neurovascular compromise must be assessed.

Case 22

Clinical details

This teenager twisted and inverted his foot while playing football. Is the lucency at the base of the fifth metatarsal a fracture or an epiphyseal line?

Radiological features

There is a fracture line and also an epiphyseal line, i.e. a horizontal fracture of the base of the fifth metatarsal and an epiphysis separated by a vertical lucency.

Diagnosis

Fracture of the base of the fifth metatarsal.

Discussion

The fracture (dashed line) and epiphyseal line (arrow) are indicated on the oblique view below (Figure 3).

Figure 3. The oblique view with the fracture outlined and the epiphyseal line indicated by an arrow.

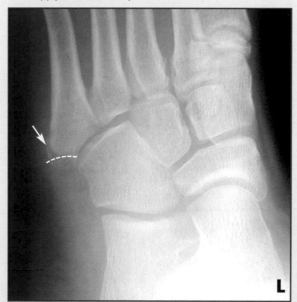

Figure 1. AP forefoot.

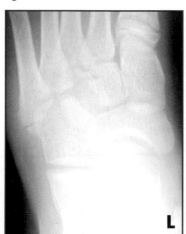

Figure 2. Oblique forefoot.

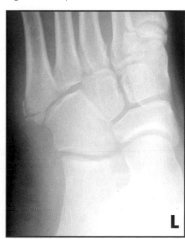

General Films

Introduction

This section does not aim to provide a comprehensive guide to general radiology, but simply demonstrates a few common medical and surgical conditions that are regularly seen at the Emergency Department, and highlights their radiological presentation.

Case I

Clinical details

This patient presented with sudden onset of breathlessness and pleuritic chest pain.

Figure I. CXR.

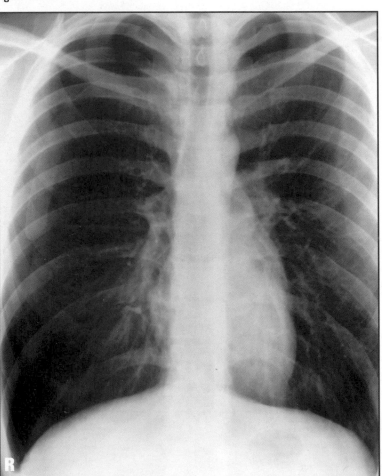

Radiological features

The right hemithorax is more radiolucent than the left side, and upon a closer look, a lung edge indicating a pneumothorax is apparent. The mediastinum is not shifted and so it is not a tension pneumothorax.

Diagnosis

Right-sided pneumothorax.

Discussion

The pneumothorax is indicated by an arrow on the chest X-ray (CXR) opposite (Figure 2).

This may be spontaneous (asthmatic) or can be associated with rib fractures and a pneumo-mediastinum (not seen here).

Figure 2. The CXR with the pneumothorax indicated by an arrow.

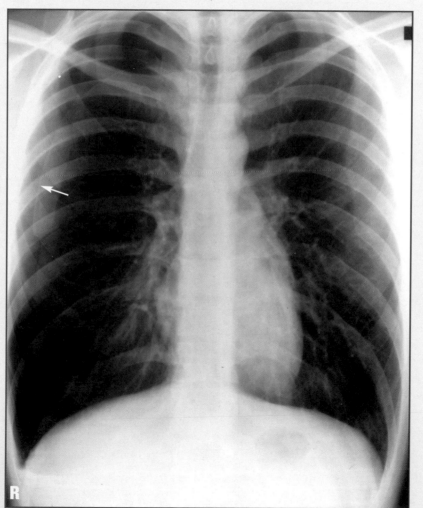

Case 2

Clinical details

This elderly patient was clammy, hypotensive and very breathless.

Figure 1. CXR.

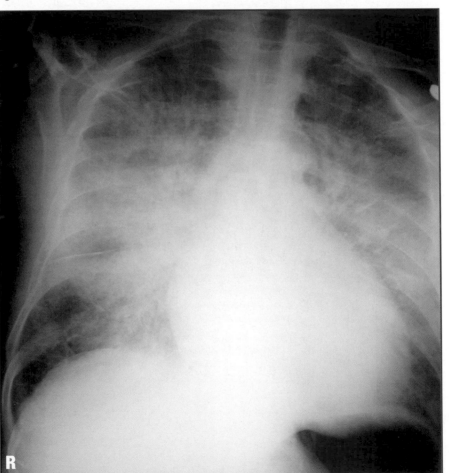

Radiological features

There is a large heart, peri-hilar haziness and increased interstitial lung markings with Kerley 'B' lines at the lung edge (horizontal thin white lines extending from the lateral edge of the lungs).

Diagnosis

Left ventricular failure.

Discussion

These are all features of pulmonary edema secondary to left ventricular failure. Kerley 'B' lines are due to fluid in the interstitial spaces (these are indicated on the CXR, Figure 2).

Figure 2. The CXR with Kerley 'B' lines indicated by an arrow.

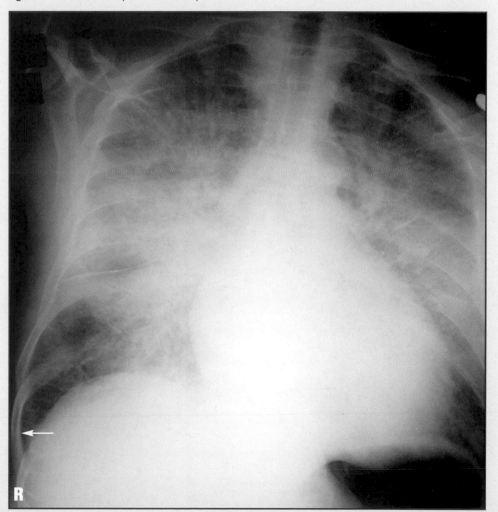

Case Studies

Case 3

Clinical details
This patient presented with a temperature and a productive cough. Is there any abnormality on the CXR?

Figure 1. CXR.

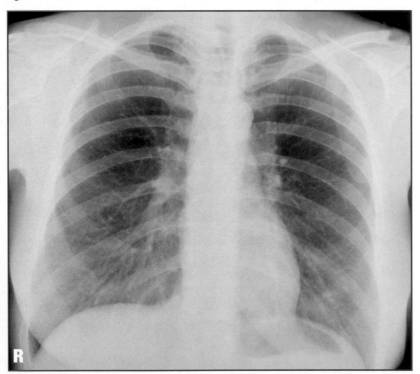

Radiological features
The lungs are clear, with no added shadowing, and the mediastinal contours look normal.

Diagnosis
Normal CXR.

Case 4

Clinical details

This young adult presented with a short history of feeling generally unwell. Nothing was found on clinical examination. Are any abnormalities evident on the CXR?

Figure 1. CXR.

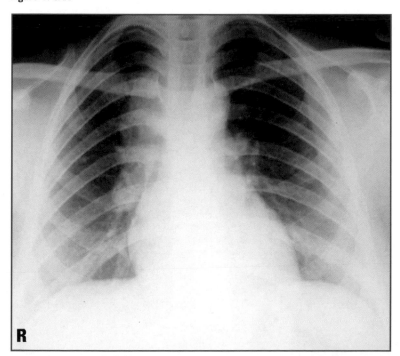

Radiological features

The right hilum is prominent, but the left is normal. This could be due to a large pulmonary artery (i.e. pulmonary artery hypertension) or lymphadenopathy. The outline is slightly lobulated suggesting lymph nodes. There is also soft-tissue shadowing adjacent to the trachea on the right (on a normal CXR, no soft-tissue shadowing is present in this area).

Diagnosis

Right para-tracheal and right hilar lymphadenopathy.

Discussion

The soft-tissue shadowing adjacent to the trachea is in fact lymphadenopathy. The most common causes of lymphadenopathy are tuberculosis, lymphoma and sarcoidosis.

Case 5

Clinical details
This patient presented with a cough that was productive of green sputum.

Figure 1. CXR.

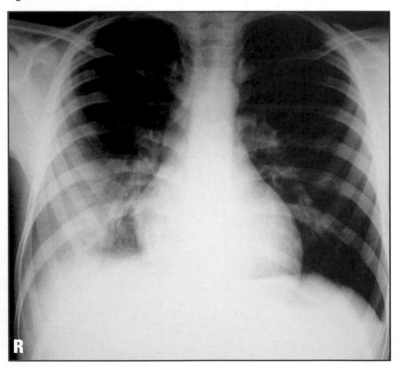

R

Radiological features
There is extra shadowing in the lung adjacent to the right hemi-diaphragm. The right heart border is seen clearly but the right hemi-diaphragm is obscured. Air bronchograms are also just visible; these are branching structures that contain air and are therefore seen as black against the white surrounding consolidation in the alveoli.

Diagnosis
Right lower lobe consolidation.

Figure 2. Magnified view of consolidation with an air bronchogram arrowed.

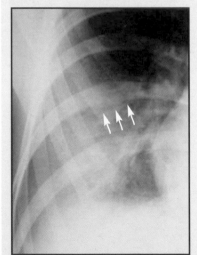

Discussion
Air bronchograms (Figure 2) are typical of consolidation (solid or liquid material in the air spaces). The most common causes include:
1. pus/inflammatory cells from infection
2. fluid from severe pulmonary edema

and more rarely:
3. blood, for example in cases of Goodpasture syndrome
4. tumor cells, for example in cases of alveolar cell carcinoma.

Case 6

Clinical details
This heavy smoker lost 2 stone in weight over a short period of time.

Figure 1. CXR.

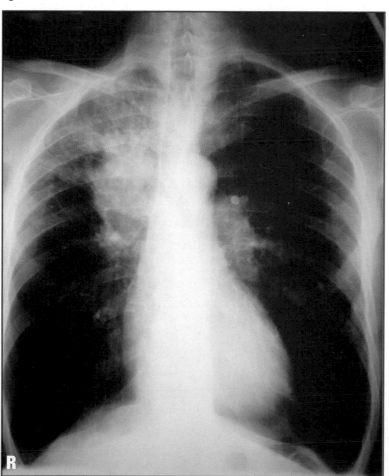

Radiological features
There is a large mass seen at the right hilum. Partial collapse of the right upper lobe is apparent as the horizontal fissure has moved upwards and consolidation is also seen within the upper lobe.

Diagnosis
Right hilar carcinoma of the lung.

Case 7

Clinical details

This patient was experiencing
severe abdominal pain.

Figure 1. CXR.

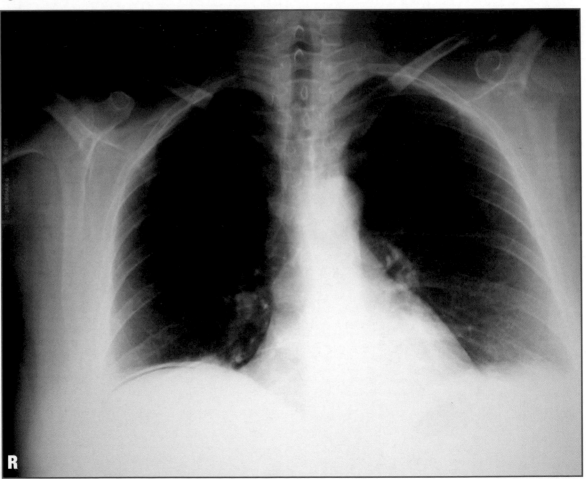

Radiological features

There is a sliver of free air under the right hemi-diaphragm above the liver on the erect CXR, indicating perforation of a gut viscus into the peritoneal cavity.

Diagnosis

Perforation.

Discussion

The sliver of free air under the right hemi-diaphragm is indicated on the CXR opposite (Figure 2).

Intra-peritoneal air is produced only when the intra-peritoneal gut is perforated. Retro-peritoneal structures, such as the third part of the duodenum, perforate into the retro-peritoneum, therefore any air released outlines retro-peritoneal structures. The most common sites of perforation are the duodenal cap (due to an ulcer) and the large bowel (due to a colonic diverticulum or carcinoma).

Figure 2. The sliver of free air under the hemi-diaphragm is indicated on the CXR (magnified view) by an arrow.

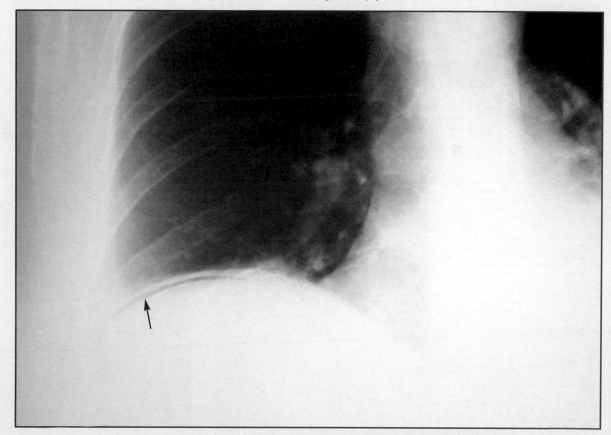

Case 8

Clinical details
These patients were experiencing
abdominal pain and constipation.
What is the abnormality in
each case?

Figure 1 (patient 8a). AP abdomen.

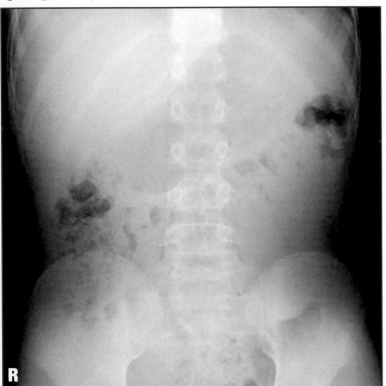

Figure 2 (patient 8b). AP abdomen.

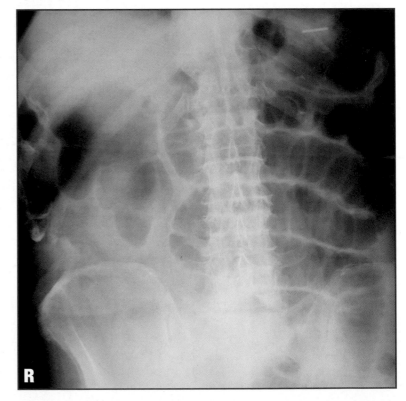

Radiological features

Patient 8a. The plain abdominal film appears normal, with no abnormality of the bowel gas pattern.

Patient 8b. The features of both small and large bowel obstruction can be seen. There are multiple loops of dilated small bowel that lie centrally with folds, which cross the entire bowel wall, i.e. they are *valvulae conniventes*. However, in the right flank, a dilated air filled caecum and ascending colon can be seen but no air-filled transverse, descending or sigmoid colon is seen. Therefore, the level of obstruction is in the ascending colon.

Diagnosis

Normal (8a) and large bowel obstruction with accompanying small bowel dilatation (8b).

Discussion

The small bowel is full of air because the ileocaecal valve is incompetent, i.e. it lets air pass back from the large bowel into the small bowel.

The radiological signs of small bowel versus large bowel obstruction are listed in Table 1.

Table 1. The radiological signs of small bowel versus large bowel obstruction.

Radiological signs	Small bowel	Large bowel
Multiple loops of bowel	Yes	Yes, if ileocaecal valve incompetent No, if ileocaecal valve competent
Single loop of dilated bowel	No	Yes
Centrally placed loops of bowel	Yes	No
Peripherally placed loops	No	Yes
Degree of dilatation	Moderate (i.e. ~ 5 cm)	Can be very dilated (i.e. ~ 8 cm)
Folds	Continuous (*valvulae conniventes*)	Incomplete (haustrae)
Common causes	Adhesions or hernias	Obstructing mass, e.g. carcinoma or diverticular mass

Case Studies

Case 9

Clinical details

This patient presented with right-sided loin to groin pain of 24 hours' duration. However, the pain had started to ease. What does the emergency intravenous urogram show?

Figure 1. Kidneys, ureter and bladder (KUB) control.

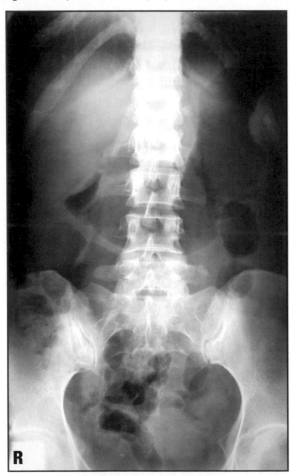

Figure 2. KUB 40 minutes after intravenous radio-opaque contrast.

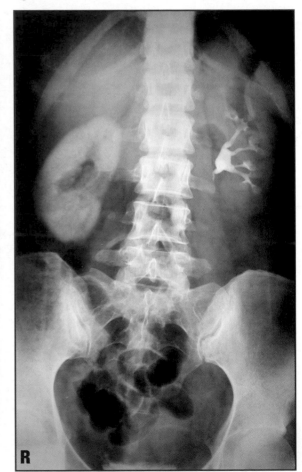

Radiological features

A calcified stone is seen in the pelvis on the control film and this was subsequently demonstrated to be within the lower ureter. After 40 minutes another film was taken, and the left kidney and left pelvicocalyceal system filled with contrast normally. On the right, there is a delayed, dense nephrogram and no filling of the right pelvicocalyceal system or ureter. The right ureteric stone eventually passed into the bladder and the obstruction was relieved.

Diagnosis

Right-sided calcified stone causing obstruction.

Discussion

The stone in the right side of the pelvis has probably recently passed down the ureter, causing renal colic and obstruction of the right side. The obstruction resolves once the stone has passed.

The calcified stone seen on the control view is indicated on Figure 3.

Figure 3. The control view with the calcified stone in the pelvis indicated by an arrow.

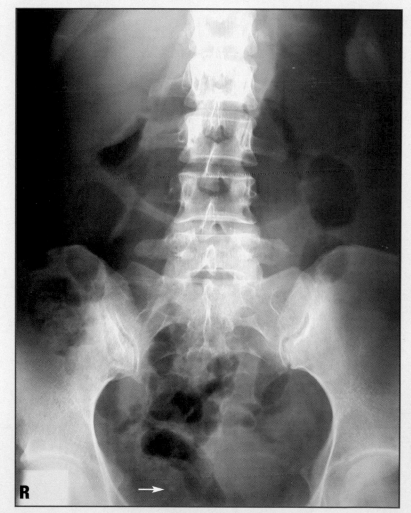

NORMAL FILMS

ABBREVIATIONS

AC	acromioclavicular		**NAI**	non-accidental injury
AP	anteroposterior		**OM**	occipitomental
ASL	anterior spinal line		**OPG**	orthopantomogram
AVN	avascular necrosis		**PA**	posteroanterior
CT	computed tomography		**PPL**	posterior pillar line
CXR	chest X-ray		**PSL**	posterior spinal line
DP	dorsoplantar		**RTA**	road traffic accident
HBL	horizontal beam lateral		**SL**	spinolaminar line
KUB	kidneys, ureter and bladder		**SMV**	submentovertical
MRI	magnetic resonance imaging		**SPL**	spinous line
MCP	metacarpophalangeal			

Index